Point of Care Testing

Editor

LINOJ SAMUEL

CLINICS IN LABORATORY MEDICINE

www.labmed.theclinics.com

Consulting Editor
MILENKO JOVAN TANASIJEVIC

June 2023 • Volume 43 • Number 2

ELSEVIER

1600 John F. Kennedy Boulevard ● Suite 1800 ● Philadelphia, Pennsylvania, 19103-2899

http://www.theclinics.com

CLINICS IN LABORATORY MEDICINE Volume 43, Number 2
June 2023 ISSN 0272-2712, ISBN-13: 978-0-443-18294-5

Editor: Taylor Hayes
Developmental Editor: Akshay Samson

Reprints. For copies of 100 or more, of articles in this publication, please contact the Commercial Reprints Department, Elsevier Inc., 360 Park Avenue South, New York, New York 10010-1710. Tel. 212-633-3874, Fax: 212-633-3820, E-mail: reprints@elsevier.com.

Clinics in Laboratory Medicine (ISSN 0272-2712) is published quarterly by Elsevier Inc., 360 Park Avenue South, New York, NY 10010-1710. Months of issue are March, June, September, and December. Business and Editorial offices: 1600 John F. Kennedy Blvd., Suite 1800, Philadelphia, PA 19103-2899. Periodicals postage paid at NewYork, NY and additional mailing offices. Subscription prices are $291.00 per year (US individuals), $657.00 per year (US institutions), $100.00 per year (US students), $374.00 per year (Canadian individuals), $798.00 per year (Canadian institutions), $100.00 per year (Canadian students), $416.00 per year (international individuals), $798.00 per year (international institutions), $185.00 (international students). Foreign air speed delivery is included in all Clinics subscription prices. All prices are subject to change without notice. POSTMASTER: Send address changes to *Clinics in Laboratory Medicine*, Elsevier Health Sciences Division, Subscription Customer Service, 3251 Riverport Lane, Maryland Heights, MO 63043. **Customer Service: 1-800-654-2452 (US). From outside of the US and Canada, call 1-314-447-8871. Fax: 1-314-447-8029. E-mail: journalscustomerservice-usa@elsevier.com (for print support) or journalsonlinesupport-usa@elsevier.com (for online support).**

Clinics in Laboratory Medicine is covered in *EMBASE/Exerpta Medica, MEDLINE/PubMed (Index Medicus), Cinahl, Current Contents/Clinical Medicine, BIOSIS and ISI/BIOMED.*

Contributors

EDITOR-IN-CHIEF

MILENKO JOVAN TANASIJEVIC, MD, MBA
Vice Chair for Clinical Pathology and Quality, Department of Pathology, Director of Clinical Laboratories, Brigham and Women's Hospital, Dana-Farber Cancer Institute, Associate Professor of Pathology, Harvard Medical School, Boston, Massachusetts, USA

EDITOR

LINOJ SAMUEL, PhD, D(ABMM)
Division Head, Clinical Microbiology, Pathology and Laboratory Medicine, Henry Ford Health, Detroit, Michigan, USA

AUTHORS

MEGAN H. AMERSON-BROWN, PhD
Assistant Professor, Department of Pathology, The University of Alabama at Birmingham, Marnix E. Heersink School of Medicine, Birmingham, Alabama, USA

ASHLEY CIMINO-MATHEWS, MD
Associate Professor, Departments of Pathology and Oncology, Johns Hopkins School of Medicine, Baltimore, Maryland, USA

LEISHA A. EMENS, MD, PhD
Professor, Department of Oncology, UPMC Hillman Cancer Center/Magee Women's Hospital, Pittsburgh, Pennsylvania, USA

ONDREJ HES, MD, PhD
Department of Pathology, Charles University in Prague, Faculty of Medicine, Plzeň University Hospital Plzeň, Pilsen, Czech Republic

GEETHA JAGANNATHAN, MBBS
Surgical Pathology Assistant, Department of Pathology, Johns Hopkins School of Medicine, Baltimore, Maryland, USA

THAER KHOURY, MD
Professor of Oncology, Pathology Department, Roswell Park Comprehensive Cancer Center, Buffalo, New York, USA

NATALIE LARSEN, MD
Resident, Department of Pathology, The University of Alabama at Birmingham, Marnix E. Heersink School of Medicine, Birmingham, Alabama, USA

MICHAEL J. LOEFFELHOLZ, PhD, D(ABMM)
Senior Director, Scientific Affairs, Cepheid, Sunnyvale, California, USA

PAUL M. LUETHY, PhD, D(ABMM)
Assistant Professor, Department of Pathology, University of Maryland School of Medicine, Baltimore, Maryland, USA

STEVEN MAHLEN, PhD, D(ABMM)
Sanford Health, Bismark, North Dakota, USA

MEHDI MANSOOR, MD, FRCPC
Department of Pathology and Laboratory Medicine, Cumming School of Medicine, University of Calgary, Rockyview General Hospital, Calgary, Alberta, Canada

LINDSEY E. NIELSEN, PhD, D(ABMM)
LN Laboratory Consulting, Nebraska, USA

ZEHRA ORDULU, MD
Department of Pathology, Immunology and Laboratory Medicine, Assistant Professor, University of Florida, Gainesville, Florida, USA

DANIEL A. ORTIZ, PhD, D(ABMM)
System Director, Microbiology and Molecular Pathology, Assistant Professor, Department of Pathology, Oakland University William Beaumont School of Medicine, Beaumont Health, Royal Oak, Michigan, USA

ASHLEIGH N. RIEGLER, PhD
Postdoctoral Fellow, Department of Pathology, The University of Alabama at Birmingham, Marnix E. Heersink School of Medicine, Birmingham, Alabama, USA

ROBERT L. SAUTTER, PhD HCLD/CC (ABB), MS, MT (ASCP), SM
RL Sautter Consulting LLC, Lancaster, South Carolina, USA

FARSHID SIADAT, MD, FRCPC
Department of Pathology and Laboratory Medicine, Cumming School of Medicine, University of Calgary, Rockyview General Hospital, Calgary, Alberta, Canada

DEENA E. SUTTER, MD, FAAP
Pediatric Infectious Disease Specialist, Tenet Physician Resources/Baptist Health System, San Antonio, Texas, USA

KIRIL TRPKOV, MD, FRCPC
Department of Pathology and Laboratory Medicine, Cumming School of Medicine, University of Calgary, Rockyview General Hospital, Calgary, Alberta, Canada

MARISSA J. WHITE, MD
Assistant Professor, Department of Pathology, Johns Hopkins School of Medicine, Baltimore, Maryland, USA

RENA R. XIAN, MD
Assistant Professor, Departments of Pathology and Oncology, Johns Hopkins School of Medicine, Baltimore, Maryland, USA

NICHOLAS YARED, MD
Infectious Disease Senior Staff, Department of Medicine, Henry Ford Health, Detroit, Michigan, USA

Contents

The Clinical Laboratory Improvement Amendments (CLIA) classifications were activated in the 1990s in partnership with the Centers for Medicare and Medicaid Services and Food and Drug Administration and included waived, moderate, and high complexity testing. The waived section of CLIA certificates allows laboratories to perform testing of analytes and methods of samples by the Food and Drug Administration. During the COVID-19 pandemic, many molecular or antigen laboratory testing methods for COVID-19 virus were quickly approved by emergency use authorization. Waived testing is now done in highly complex, moderately complex, and waived testing laboratories, and some at-home testing.

The practical challenges of point-of-care testing (POCT) include analytical performance and quality compared with testing performed in a central laboratory and higher cost per test compared with laboratory-based tests. These challenges can be addressed with new test technology, consensus, and practice guidelines for the use of POCT, instituting a quality management system and data connectivity in the POCT setting, and studies that demonstrate evidence of clinical and economic value of POCT.

Before the molecular age, cell culture was the gold standard for confirmatory diagnosis of viral and atypical infectious diseases. Typical cell culture methodologies are costly, require days (or weeks) for results, and require significant technical expertise. As a result, cell culture is impractical for timely diagnostic testing in most of the health care environments. Traditional bacterial culture methods, also have disadvantages due to the need for incubation, subsequent identification of pathogens, and significant technical expertise. This article discusses the general considerations of antigen and molecular assays and the merits and factors to consider when implementing diagnostic assays for several common pathogens.

Diagnostics for particular populations outside of traditional health care settings have driven development of point-of-care testing (POCT). POCT is particularly suitable for patients with infections conditions to mitigate infection spread via its provision in venues with less concern for stigma. Patients in rural or resource-limited settings can benefit from POCT through more timely diagnosis and linkage-to-care. However, gaps in POCT availability compared with better-resourced, urban counterparts persist. Leveraging communication technologies, using mobile clinics, changing national health care policy, and implementing novel geospatial science concepts can address limitations of POCT use and reduce POCT access gaps in these settings.

Point-of-care testing for sexually transmitted infections is essential for controlling transmission and preventing sequelae in high-risk populations. Since the World Health Organization published the ASSURED criteria, point-of-care testing has improved for use in large population screening and rapid testing that prevents loss of clinical follow-up. Recent advancements have been advantageous for low-resource areas allowing testing at a minimal cost without reliable electricity or refrigeration. Point-of-care nucleic acid detection and amplification techniques are recommended, but are often inaccessible in low-resource areas. Future advancements in point-of-care diagnostic testing should focus on improving antibody-based assays, monitoring viral loads, and detecting antimicrobial resistance.

Invasive fungal infections are increasing worldwide due to factors such as climate change and immunomodulating therapies. Unfortunately, the detection of these infections is limited due to the low sensitivity and long periods required for laboratory testing. Point-of-care testing could lead to more rapid diagnosis of these often devasting infections. However, there are currently no true point-of-care tests on the market for the detection of fungi. In this article, the current state of fungal antigen and molecular testing is reviewed, with commentary on the potential for development and use in the point-of-care setting.

Hot Topics in Cancer Testing and New Developments

Metaplastic breast carcinoma (MpBC) is a heterogeneous group of tumors that clinically could be divided into low risk and high risk. It is important to recognize the different types of MpBC, as the high-risk subtypes have worse clinical outcomes than triple-negative breast cancer. It is important for the pathologist to be aware of the MpBC entities and use the proposed algorithms (morphology and immunohistochemistry) to assist in rendering the final diagnosis. Few pitfalls are discussed, including misinterpretation of immunohistochemistry and certain histomorphologies, particularly spindle lesions associated with complex sclerosing lesions.

This article focuses on the recent advances in ovarian sex cord–stromal tumors, predominantly in the setting of their molecular underpinnings. The integration of genetic information with morphologic and immunohistochemical findings in this rare subset of tumors is of clinical significance from refining the diagnostic and prognostic stratifications to genetic counseling.

This review summarizes current knowledge on several novel and emerging renal entities, including eosinophilic solid and cystic renal cell carcinoma (RCC), RCC with fibromyomatous stroma, anaplastic lymphoma kinase-rearranged RCC, low-grade oncocytic renal tumor, eosinophilic vacuolated tumor, thyroidlike follicular RCC, and biphasic hyalinizing psammomatous RCC. Their clinical features, gross and microscopic morphology, immunohistochemistry, and molecular and genetic features are described. The diagnosis of most of them rests on recognizing their morphologic features using immunohistochemistry. Accurate diagnosis of these entitles will further reduce the category of "unclassifiable renal carcinomas/tumors" and will lead to better clinical management and improved patient prognostication.

Predictive biomarker testing on metastatic breast cancer is essential for determining patient eligibility for targeted therapeutics. The National Comprehensive Cancer Network currently recommends assessment of specific biomarkers on metastatic tumor subtypes, including hormone receptors, HER2, and BRCA1/2 mutations, on all newly metastatic breast cancers subtypes; programmed death-ligand 1 on metastatic triple-negative carcinomas; and PIK3CA mutation status on estrogen receptor-positive carcinomas. In select circumstances mismatch repair protein deficiency and/or microsatellite insufficiency, tumor mutation burden, and NTRK translocation status are also testing options. Novel biomarker testing, such as detecting PIK3CA mutations in circulating tumor DNA, is expanding in this rapidly evolving arena.

CLINICS IN LABORATORY MEDICINE

SERIES OF RELATED INTEREST

Advances in Molecular Pathology
Available at: https://www.journals.elsevier.com/advances-in-molecular-pathology

---

THE CLINICS ARE NOW AVAILABLE ONLINE!
Access your subscription at:
www.theclinics.com

Preface

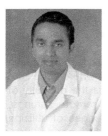

Linoj Samuel, PhD
Editor

In this issue of *Clinics in Laboratory Medicine*, the focus is on the increasing role of point-of-care (POC) testing in patient care and management. In a previous issue before the onset of the COVID-19 pandemic, Samuel and colleagues[1] commented on the growing importance of POC testing and the need for appropriate oversight. The COVID-19 pandemic put an unprecedented strain on diagnostic laboratories across the world. Traditional centralized laboratory-based diagnostic testing was challenged by severe shortages in the supply chain. The unprecedented demand for testing coupled with supply and staffing challenges resulted in significant delays in time to results.[2] This opened a unique window of opportunity for POC-based testing to fill the gap.

POC testing offered the possibility of both rapid turnaround time and near-patient testing with the use of limited resources. However, the initial use of POC testing during the COVID-19 pandemic was marred by substandard products. The regulatory framework in the United States early during the pandemic was also challenged by its inability to respond to the changing needs. The early restrictions placed by the public health emergency and the emergency use authorization initially limited the ability of laboratories to implement COVID-19 testing. Subsequent changes brought about by the advancing pandemic swung the pendulum too far in the opposite direction and resulted in release of POC test kits that had poor sensitivity and/or specificity.[3] Toward the end of the pandemic, we saw increased availability and acceptance of the use of POC tests not only in the clinical setting but also in the at-home setting. Patients were increasingly more comfortable with self-collection of the samples and the convenience of testing in the privacy of their own homes. In addition, the pandemic accelerated the development of molecular-based POC test kits. POC molecular-based testing are now widely available in the clinical setting, and even at-home molecular POC test kits are now available. These advances may help address the performance concerns related to POC testing, but significant challenges remain.

In this issue, Dr Robert Sautter addresses the regulatory challenges during the COVID-19 pandemic and the subsequent impact on the testing landscape. Drs Ortiz and Loeffelholz in turn address the practical challenges of implementing POC testing

Clin Lab Med 43 (2023) ix–x
https://doi.org/10.1016/j.cll.2023.04.001
0272-2712/23/© 2023 Published by Elsevier Inc.

in the clinical setting. Careful consideration needs to be given to all aspects of testing from location to personnel. Dr Nielsen and colleagues examine whether the accelerated development of molecular POC testing means that antigen testing with its related challenges will remain relevant.

The advances made during this pandemic are not limited to COVID-19 alone, and improved POC testing has the potential to significantly change how we detect and manage diseases caused by a number of different pathogens and in a variety of clinical settings. Dr Yared evaluates the impact of POC testing for specific populations, in particular, for HIV and HCV testing, and also in remote/rural settings where access to traditional laboratory testing can be challenging. He also addresses the difficulty of maintaining quality control even for CLIA-waived POC testing in remote settings. Along similar lines, Dr Riegler and colleagues assessed the challenges of utilizing POC testing to target sexually transmitted infections (STI) in resource-poor settings. While molecular-based assays are the preferred test of choice for STI, the limited availability of such tests requires the use of antigen-based testing in some scenarios. Both Drs Yared and Riegler comment on the need not just for better-quality POC tests but also for a broader test menu that targets more pathogens, targets resistance markers, and when appropriate, is even able to provide quantitative viral loads. Finally, Dr Luethy reviews the lack of POC testing options for fungal pathogens. The impact of climate change is manifested in the increased geographic range and incidence of a variety of fungal diseases. In the absence of easily accessible testing capabilities, we will struggle to contain the spread of these pathogens.

Looking beyond COVID-19, the authors together make the case for a concerted effort to push the envelope with POC testing. We need better-performing tests that target a wide range of pathogens and even resistance markers to facilitate early appropriate therapy. We also need better accessibility of tests allowing even at-home testing where needed. And if that happens, we need to develop processes that allow us to monitor the quality of at-home testing and incorporate those results into the continuum of care.

Linoj Samuel, PhD
Clinical Microbiology
Pathology and Laboratory Medicine
Henry Ford Health
2799 West Grand Boulevard
Detroit, MI 48202, USA

E-mail address:
lsamuel2@hfhs.org

REFERENCES

1. Linoj Samuel. Point-of-Care Testing in Microbiology. Clin Lab Med 2020;40(4):483–94. Available at: https://pubmed.ncbi.nlm.nih.gov/33121617/.
2. Leber AL, Peterson E, Bard JD, et al. The Hidden Crisis in the Times of COVID-19: Critical Shortages of Medical Laboratory Professionals in Clinical Microbiology. J Clin Microbiol 2022;60(8):e0024122. Available at: https://pubmed.ncbi.nlm.nih.gov/35658527/.
3. Truong TT, Bard JD, Butler-Wu SM. Rapid antigen assays for SARS-CoV-2: Promise and peril. Clin Lab Med 2022;42(2): 203–22. Available at: https://www.ncbi.nlm.nih.gov/pmc/articles/PMC8894733/.

Regulatory Approach to Point-of-Care/At-Home Testing in the United States

Robert L. Sautter, PhD HCLD/CC (ABB), MS, MT (ASCP), SM

KEYWORDS

- Point-of-care testing • CMS (Centers for Medicare and Medicaid Services)
- COVID-19 testing • CLIA (Clinical Laboratory Improvement Amendments)
- Guidelines • Waived and home testing

KEY POINTS

- A huge benefit to laboratory testing occurred in 1988 and the 1990s resulting in more rapid results and improving patient care.
- Classification of laboratory tests as waived, moderate, and high complexity allowing for personnel responsible for performing tests, regulations including testing, oversight, and levels of complex and simplified testing laboratory classifications.
- Performing waived testing in the near patient setting with appropriate oversight to ensure accurate results.
- Modification of regulations to allow home-based testing and appropriate confirmatory testing.
- Consequences of failing to follow testing guidelines and possible effect on patient well-being.

INTRODUCTION

Laboratory testing is extremely important in diagnosing diseases and treating patients. It is arguably involved in 70% of medical diagnoses.[1–5] The accuracy and speed of results is important to accurately treat patients.[4,5] Until recently many nonlaboratory health care providers did not realize how important laboratory tests were and did not follow up with quality control, quality assurance, and training. Therefore the results were often questionable and could result in putting patients at risk.[1,5] During the most recent pandemic (COVID-19) it has become apparent that laboratory testing and accurate results are paramount to good patient care.[6] Results of important laboratory tests are often delayed because of the transport of samples to the core laboratory or reference laboratory. A multidisciplinary team is needed to institute laboratory testing, and it is important for the laboratory to lead and be part of this team.[5–9] These teams should discuss the advantages and disadvantages of performing tests either in the main laboratory or in

RL Sautter Consulting LLC, Lancaster, SC 29720, USA
E-mail address: sautterfamily@hotmail.com

Clin Lab Med 43 (2023) 145–154
https://doi.org/10.1016/j.cll.2023.02.001
labmed.theclinics.com
0272-2712/23/© 2023 Elsevier Inc. All rights reserved.

the point of care (near patient testing) (POC).[5,7–10] Many things must be considered before approving tests for the laboratory: adequately trained technologists, directors that have expertise and knowledge in the laboratory of the new tests, the technology that is currently available, and support of nonlaboratory health care workers and physicians. Administration should also be on board with the testing offered. In particular, when complex testing, such as molecular testing, is being brought on board, several things mentioned previously must be considered.[4,5,8] This is an important task but is even more difficult when the testing is only approved by Emergency Use Authorization (EUA) and there are no standard Food and Drug Administration (FDA) comparisons and guidelines for preuse evaluation and comparisons with standard methods. This would mean that no standard approval or complex evaluation of the tests are performed as required by FDA before the pandemic.

HISTORY

POC testing has been active since ancient Egyptian times.[1,2] In the last 30 years it has become an important part of diagnosing diseases.[5] In particular, in 1988 the Clinical Laboratory Improvement Amendments (CLIA) were outlined to help classify laboratory tests and also to oversee the testing process.[1,3–5] Before this amendment, testing outside of the core laboratory was not regulated, which led to inaccurate results that put patients at risk.[1,4–8] Even after the institution of these guidelines, the testing personnel and laboratory directors did not follow testing guidelines and therefore many errors occurred in the results.[1,5] Following the waived testing study[1] the institution of inspections and following quality guidelines and manufacturer's instructions for waived testing as outlined by the companies that manufactured the tests was determined to be a problem in inaccurate testing.[1,5,8] Although it was concerning that health care workers and physicians would not follow laboratory guidelines and manufacturer's procedures, the general public with "at-home" testing may or may not follow good laboratory testing.[1,4,5]

The evaluation of waived laboratory testing over the years has proven that many testing sites do not follow guidelines, perform required QC/QA, or training or oversight of the testing personnel.[1,4] The waived laboratories must follow the most stringent requirements by either the state that they are in or the federal requirements. Some states accept federal requirements and others have more stringent guidelines. However, until laboratory inspections occurred in waived laboratories, errors were rampant and the process did not improve.[1,4]

During the worldwide COVID-19 pandemic the need for laboratory tests and availability for testing was off the charts. Testing started in the federal and state government laboratories and then went to academic medical centers. The need became so great that testing was increased across the United States with many sites performing testing including reference laboratories, small hospitals, physician offices, and drive-through sites for collection. The need was so great that millions of tests were being done and approval of new tests was required. The EUA was instituted during the COVID-19 pandemic and a total of 439 EUA tests were approved for use. This stimulated a concern about proper testing and training became a legitimate problem because many medical laboratory scientists became overworked and exhausted. With the numbers of laboratory workers already becoming difficult to recruit, POC and at-home testing became an option. Accuracy of testing is also of concern with at-home testing and testing at multiple sites in the population.

The number of laboratories and the numbers of waived tests have increased dramatically (**Fig. 1**). Waived testing laboratories are by far the highest number of laboratories in

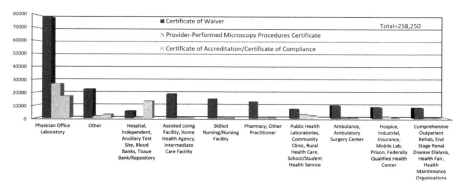

Fig. 1. US laboratory demographics, June 2017. (Data obtained from CMS Quality Improvement & evaluation System (QIES) database, 06/27/2017. Laboratory types in QIES data are self-reported. Numbers included laboratories in CLIA-exempt states of NY and WA. Data do not include CLIA certificate of registration laboratories. Anderson N, Stang H. Promoting good laboratory practices for waived infectious disease and provide-performed microscopy testing. Clin Microbiol Newsl 2017; 39:183-8.).

the United States with most of them having a CLIA waived certificate (see **Fig. 1**; **Fig. 2**).[1,5] They have grown immensely over the years.[1,4,5,10] The federal guidelines for testing in waived laboratories are much less stringent than nonwaived laboratories (**Table 1**). In addition, the number of analytes has also grown.[1,4,5,10]

Most waived laboratories use rapid antigen detection tests (RADT) for detection of infectious diseases. Typically these rapid tests are not sensitive and are typically dependent on and more reliable when the patient is demonstrating symptoms of the disease.[11] If they are tested without symptoms, the positive predictive value of their results is less than 50% even if the specificity of the test is 98%.[12] They are also dependent on the incidence of the disease in the population tested; with an incidence of 1% and a specificity of 98%, the positive predictive value would be 28.8%. This means that out of every 100 positive samples, close to 71.2% would be false positives.[11] This outlines why these positive tests should be confirmed with a more accurate test, such as molecular tests. If the incidence of the disease is high in the population and the patient has symptoms, the false-positive rate is much lower.[11]

Despite the nuances of mass testing, RADT used in Europe showed a decrease in active cases in spite of the parameters mentioned previously.[11] At-home testing of RADT was performed in the United Kingdom and the United States. Data from at-home testing show a significant decrease in sensitivity determined during testing by health care workers and the untrained performing testing, 70% to 77.8% in research and health care workers compared with 57.7% of untrained at-home testers.[11] At-home collection of swabs showed that only 80% of those collected were performed by clinicians.[13,14] The storage of the test kits can affect the sensitivity of the results.[11]

With the need for high-capacity testing during the COVID-19 pandemic, molecular testing has been approved for POC testing and possibly at-home testing. A more sensitive alternative, rapid molecular testing, is a possibility with high throughput. Rapid COVID waived testing does not really have a rapid throughput with a large number of samples and usually only tests for COVID.

Centers for Medicare and Medicaid Services (CMS) updated their guidance (October 7, 2022) on some of these concerning POC or inpatient care settings molecular and antigen testing requirements for certified laboratories performing FDA-approved EUA tests.[15] These antigen and molecular tests were approved under the

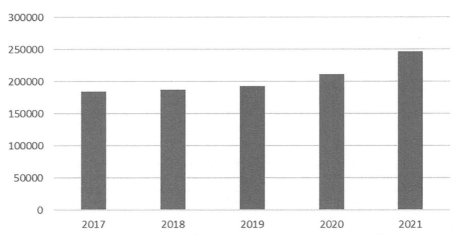

Fig. 2. The rise of certified waived laboratories and analytes "The Rise of POC Testing". (*Data from* CLIA Historical Numbers – January 2022. https://www.cms.gov/Regulations-and-Guidance/Legislation/CLIA/Downloads/2021-1993_Historical_Numbers.pdf.)

EUA to be performed and requested by health care providers after onset of symptoms. CMS does not approve testing of patients that does not follow these guidelines, in particular those laboratories under the CLIA 1988 certificates and testing patients that are asymptomatic.[15] They must follow the instructions for use by the manufacturer.[15] Also, nonwaived laboratories must establish performance of the system before reporting patient results.[15]

COVID POINT-OF-CARE AND HOME TESTING

During the COVID pandemic testing had begun under EUA approved by the FDA. This outbreak was classified as COVID-19 and was caused by COVID-2 released from Wuhan, China. Many tests used in state and federal laboratories and core and reference laboratories were laboratory-developed tests. In a short period of time tests were

Table 1
The regulations for waived and nonwaived laboratories for POC and at-home testing[3]

Requirement	Waived	Nonwaived
Personnel	No requirement	Testing and leadership must have appropriate degree and training
Quality	Must follow manufactures' instructions	The laboratory must have a quality program
Proficiency testing	No requirement	External or alternative proficiency testing for all tests
Safety	No requirement	Safety procedures are required
Validation and verification	No requirement	Requirement
Enforcement	None	Biennial inspections
At-home testing	With approval	NA (Not Applicable)

available for other smaller laboratories and they were available from manufacturers, the numbers of which have exploded and EUA approval for COVID testing happened quickly. Millions of tests were performed in certified and accredited laboratories.[13,14] The testing was divided by the methods and analytes were approved to be used in high complexity, moderate complexity, and waived laboratories.[14,16] The total number of laboratories has increased. In September of 2022, the laboratory types are: certificate type (nonexempt only) compliance 17,708; waiver 243,951; provider performed microscopy 27,257; and accreditation 16,039.[17]

As of September 27, 2022, more than 430 COVID-19 tests have been approved for EUAs.[18] In this communication the director of the federal center for devices and radiologic health, stated that laboratory testing is key to combating the COVID-19 pandemic and if further methods of testing is required, that instead of approving them through EUA they should be approved using traditional premarket approval of these tests. "All tests for covid with molecular, antigen testing, and serology were approved for use in the laboratories in the United States."[18]

However, it also states that,[18]

"Moving forward, the FDA generally intends to focus its review on EUA requests and supplemental EUA requests from experienced developers for and not focus on at home testing but rather focus on the items below.

- Diagnostic tests that are likely to have a significant benefit to public health (such as those that employ new technologies);
- Diagnostic tests that are likely to fulfill an unmet need (such as diagnosing infection with a new variant or subvariant);
- Supplemental EUA requests for previously authorized tests when the request is intended to fulfill a condition of authorization or includes a modification that will significantly benefit public health or fulfill an unmet need; and
- Tests for which the EUA request is from (or supported by) a U.S. government stakeholder, such as tests funded by the Biomedical Advanced Research and Development Authority (BARDA) or the National Institutes of Health's Rapid Acceleration of Diagnostics (RADx)."

The federal administration has made available 350 million COVID tests to the public and delivered to their homes.[19] Although this allows most Americans access to testing, it does not do anything to ensure these tests will be done accurately.[1,4,5] There is no need for a physician's order for the test, no training of the testing individuals, no follow-up for either positive or negative tests, no capture of data to track the test results, and no pretest probability for the reliability of the test results. Although at-home tests do offer an avenue for the public to get testing done, it may not give accurate data to the family, their physician, or infection control and epidemiology.

Positives in Health Care for Doing Point-of-Care Testing

Some of the obvious advantages to POC testing are (1) rapid results, laboratory results available while the patient is evaluated by care givers; (2) current testing methods (NAAT [Nucleic Acid Amplification Test] and improved antigen testing) are robust and are sensitive and accurate; (3) some NAAT POC testing methods are now comparable with those methods offered in the core laboratory (https://www.cdc.gov/cliac/past-meetings.html); and (4) these are similar tests to sexually transmissible diseases, group A streptococcus, and some urine tests that clinics and physician's offices are used to running.[20]

Home test advantages are they allow families to test those that are sick and then distance them from their families if positive and if negative to not modify their activities, and they give caregivers reason to expedite office visits for a positive patient. Negative antigen tests in symptomatic patients and positive antigen tests in asymptomatic patients are recommended to be confirmed with a NAAT test "Given rapid tests' lower sensitivities and specificities, it's a good idea to use a PCR tests to confirm positive antigen tests in asymptomatic individuals and negative antigen tests in symptomatic individuals, as well as close contacts of positive cases. A PCR test can act as a 'second opinion'." [21]

Possible Negatives of Performing Point-of-Care Testing

There some obvious negatives of performing COVID testing at the POC.[20] The overall cost of performing testing at the POC is a negative. Both reagent cost and the cost of instrumentation is high. This is why administration must be behind bringing the testing to multiple sites because the cost of running multiple sites with the same testing is large, so confirmation of the need to do this is extremely important. Another negative is that most of the testing at POC contains limited analytes.

Some challenges with POC include test performance by nonlaboratory personnel without training and guidance.[4] Quality concerns for waived laboratory testing includes: lack of training in testing and quality assessment, constant turnover of employees, and a total lack of personnel training. Strategies to address these concerns include administrative structure for organization and oversight before instituting testing. A laboratory stewardship team to oversee POC testing for good quality results is of utmost importance.[4,5,9] This is extremely important to address, training, constant oversight, following procedures, and maintaining procedure manuals (manufactures procedures), taking into account preanalytical, analytical, and postanalytical parameters to allow good samples, testing, and data management.[4,5] The flu variant of 2009 H1N1 actually was detected with higher sensitivity using DFA (Direct Flourescent Antibody) and polymerase chain reaction when respiratory cells were detected in the sample at levels of greater than 60.[22,23]

At-home testing during COVID showed a rise in the numbers tested and also opens up questions about its reliability and future of testing and diagnosing infectious diseases (discussed next).

THE FUTURE OF POINT-OF-CARE, NEAR PATIENT TESTING, AND AT-HOME TESTING

The future of POC and near patient testing is using evaluated test methods and following the guidelines for waived, moderate, and high complexity testing depending on the laboratory classification. Under the waived CLIA certificate, these sites will be following guidelines from state and federal guidelines. Those testing in laboratories will adhere to the current guidelines. Some things that must be concentrated on are found in Sautter and colleagues[5]:

- Managing College of American Pathologists, The Joint Commission, COLA, and CLIA inspections at the POC
- Turning nonlaboratorians into testing personnel
- Competency assessment and education
- Quality control, handling failures and review
- Managing outpatient clinics and family practice centers
- Gaining physician and nursing allies
- Evaluating new instrumentation and justification
- Controlling how POC testing gets into the facility
- Challenges of data management

In particular the management of testing during a pandemic is certainly contentious. We have seen this over the years; an example is the H1N1 outbreak of 2009, the largest viral pandemic outbreak in 40 years in 2009.[5,22]

An evaluation of testing done during the H1N1 outbreak in New York showed that the sensitivity of antigen tests for the variant flu virus was 17.8%.[11,24] The current testing for flu at the time was not adequate to detect the organism. Also questions about the sample type ideal for detection of the virus was also raised.[22] It is not unusual for pathogenic viruses to change with an antigenic drift that changes the virus minimally, this occurs with flu viruses and can change them enough that second infections can occur in a person that was previously infected.[25] However antigenic drift can also occur and is mostly associated with pandemic flu, such as H1N1.[25]

During the COVID-19 pandemic five waves and three variants occurred over time and resulted in changes in infectivity and severity. These changes are called lineages of the virus (genetic variations).[26]

At-home testing opens many questions about reliability and concerns of the need and whether they will help the patient (eg, did they have symptoms, did their caregiver suggest testing, and many others). However, the White House memo discussed later seems much more reasonable. Including education of patients and providers has expanded the testing for COVID.

The institution of sending millions of COVID tests out to the public and not requiring potential patients to report the result can be worrisome. During this time of many hundred types of tests approved by EUA, it is almost impossible to capture the results of POC and home testing to assess the incidence of disease. Putting the testing results, immunology rates, and mortality rates into data files and sharing this with government leaders and health care professionals while keeping staff safe during these pandemics is an extremely important postanalytical phase of testing.[9]

One laboratory-developed test from the Centers for Disease Control and Prevention was available in about 2 months from the start of the outbreak and available to state health departments and large health care organizations; manufacturers' testing was available many months later. There were no EUA approvals for testing in health care settings or home testing, such as was available for the COVID outbreak. Evaluation of other viral detection methods (DFA, antigen testing, culture, and others) had to be evaluated by the laboratories to make sure they could detect the H1N1 variant.[27]

With the start of laboratory testing for COVID-19 many tests were EUA-approved and also some were approved for POC and in-home testing. Antigen tests are not as sensitive and robust as molecular tests. As the virus mutated and produced other variants, the likelihood of being able to detect the disease was in question.[11]

SUMMARY

The COVID-19 outbreak and pandemic resulted in many more deaths and infections across the world compared with recent viral infections. It became and still is a danger during a contentious time in the world in general. Testing was brought to laboratories in the United States as soon as possible with no manufacturer's approval from standard FDA evaluations. The speed at which testing was done was amazing and eventually resulted in hundreds of tests available for serology, antigen testing, and molecular NAAT. Under the previous and current White House leadership COVID testing and vaccinations became available much faster than previous H1N1 vaccines and testing.[22] This was achieved using an EUA and was done when no approved alternatives were available.[9] The Centers for Disease Control and Prevention and state public health laboratories, as they did for H1N1 testing, began testing for COVID-19. Unlike the H1N1 outbreak, where no EUA approval was instituted, testing for COVID was started following EUA by large reference laboratories, academic centers, and private large hospital systems.[7] This testing expanded into hundreds of thousands of tests each day, in addition to many POC sites across the country. It is clear now the importance of laboratory tests and medical laboratory scientists in making disease diagnosis.[9,17] Good laboratory practices must be followed, especially during a deadly pandemic, such as COVID. Diagnostic management teams, laboratory stewardship, and laboratory technology teams are needed to choose accurate testing methods.[1,5] Some of the most important parameters are the preanalytical, analytical, and postanalytical test phases.[5] There is a need to focus on all phases of testing. Of concern is that 70% of laboratory errors are associated with preanalytical errors.[1,3,5,6,8,9]

Testing in the future is discussed in an FDA news release.[18] Although the FDA is suggesting review of new tests using a 510K evaluation, they also think that some EUA approvals may also occur. When changes in the wave of infections with variants of the virus occur then new testing may be needed. To date five waves of infections have occurred and three variants have been seen in the United States. The most transmissible variant is the Omicron variant. Fortunately, the Omicron variant does not have the high mortality rate that previous variants had but is very communicable and has quickly spread throughout the United States. The institution of vaccines, therapy, and laboratory testing has aided the health care field in battling this pandemic.

A recent White House memo states that: "The nation's testing supply has increased dramatically. We now have free testing sites at 21,500 locations around the country. In January 2021, there were no rapid, at-home tests on the market available to Americans; during January 2022, there were more than 480 million at-home tests available to Americans on top of all other testing options."[28] In addition, in-home testing must be regulated and not be done with millions of tests sent to the general public for use. This was and is a concerning approach to testing and monitoring the population. No control or training was done and no data were available from most of this testing. The Federal government and administration has mentioned that updates and guidance will be available. "The Administration will put forth new educational efforts for the public and providers so that Americans can rapidly access treatments. The Administration will establish 'One-Stop Test to Treat' locations at pharmacy-based clinics, community health centers, Long-Term Care Facilities, and the U.S. Department of Veterans Affairs (VA) facilities across the country. 'One-stop' sites will be operational by March."[28]

It is unclear what will be available in the future for COVID testing or reacting to another pandemic. However, after going through two enormous pandemics over the last 10 to 13 years (H1N1 and COVID-19) we are much more prepared for another outbreak and could respond in several different ways. As the White House memo states, "As the country emerges from the Omicron wave, our path forward relies on maintaining and continually enhancing the numerous tools we now have to protect ourselves and our loved ones–from vaccines, to tests, to treatments, to masks, and more."

One can only hope that we will be prepared for any new viral pandemic or for variants of the COVID-19 infections. We must learn from our history (quick testing platforms, vaccinations manufactured, distribution of vaccines, and recruiting and listening to laboratorians about the critical needs for this specialty)[29]; we must remember from 2009 to the present to protect our population from serious infections.

CLINICS CARE POINTS

- Follow Best Practices During Testing: The Pre-analytic phase, Test orders, Patient identification, Pretest instructions and information, Specimen collection and handling.
- The Analytic Phase, Quality Control (QC), Test Performance, Results Interpretation.
- Resolving problems; The Post-analytic phase :Reporting Test Results, Confirmatory testing, Maintaining records of referred testing [23].

DISCLOSURE

The author currently consults and has recently received payment for services from the following companies: Abbott Laboratories, Alere, Talis Biomedical Corporation, Madison Core Labs, and Affinity Biosensors. No funding was obtained for this article.

REFERENCES

1. Anderson N, Stang H. Promoting good laboratory practices for waived infectious disease and provider-performed microscopy testing. Clin Microbiol Newsl 2017; 39:183–8.
2. Kricka LJ, Park JY, Reprish A, et al. The evolution and future of point-of-care testing. Point Care 2015;14:110–5.
3. Hallworth MJ. The 70% claim: what is the evidence base? Ann Clin Biochem 2011;48:487–8.
4. Sautter RL, Lipford EH. Point-of-care testing: guidelines and challenges. N C Med J 2007;68:132–5.
5. Sautter RL, Earnest DM, Halstead DC. What's old is new again: laboratory oversight of point of care testing—guidelines, challenges, and practical strategies. Clin Microbiol Newsl 2018;40:191–7.
6. Sogbesan K, Sogbesan T, Hata DJ, et al. Use of self-collected saliva samples for the detection of SARS-CoV-2. Lab Med 2022;lmac051. https://doi.org/10.1093/labmed/lmac051.
7. Snyder J. and Sautter RL, Evolving role of the laboratory: practical information on the laboratory and COVID-19. Hosting by science repository, Science Repository, 2020, doi:10.31487/j.JCMCR.2020.03.04, previously published in Available at: https://bit.ly/3iLw9bJ. Accessed March 9, 2023.
8. Miller JM, Binnicker MJ, Campbell S, et al. A guide to utilization of the microbiology laboratory for diagnosis of infectious diseases: 2018 update by the Infectious Diseases Society of America and the American Society for Microbiology. Clin Infect Dis 2018;67(6):e1–94.
9. Halstead DC, Sautter RL. New paradigm, new opportunities: laboratory stewardship. Clin Microbiol Newsl 2018;40:175–80.
10. CLSI. Point-of-care testing for infectious diseases. 1st edition. Wayne (PA): Clinical and Laboratory Standards Institute; 2020. CLSI report POCT15.
11. Truong TT, Dien Bard J, Butler-Wu SM. Rapid antigen assays for SARS-CoV-2: promise and peril. Clin Lab Med 2022;42(2):203–22.
12. Tenny S. and Hoffman MR. Prevalence. [Updated 2022 may 24]. In: StatPearls [internet]. Treasure island (FL): StatPearls publishing, Available at: https://www.ncbi.nlm.nih.gov/books/NBK430867/, 2022. Accessed March 9, 2023.

13. McCulloch DJ, Kim AE, Wilcox NC, et al. Comparison of unsupervised home self-collected midnasal swabs with clinician-collected nasopharyngeal swabs for detection of SARS-CoV-2 infection. JAMA Netw Open 2020;3(7):e20163.
14. Rader B, Gertz A, Iuliano AD, et al. Use of at-home COVID-19 tests—United States, August 23, 2021–March 12, 2022. MMWR Morb Mortal Wkly Rep 2022;71:489–94.
15. Updated CLIA SARS-CoV-2 molecular and antigen point of care test enforcement discretion. Available at: https://www.cms.gov/files/document/clia-sars-cov-2-point-care-test-enforcement-discretion.pdf. Accessed 10/16/2022.
16. CLIA statistical tables/graphs. Available at: https://www.cms.gov/Regulations-and-Guidance/Legislation/CLIA/CLIA_Statistical_Tables_Graphs. Accessed 10/16/2022.
17. Categorization of tests. Available at: https://www.cms.gov/Regulations-and-Guidance/Legislation/CLIA/Categorization_of_Tests. Accessed 10/16/2022.
18. Coronavirus (COVID-19) update: FDA updates COVID -19 test policy, encourages developers to seek traditional premarket review for most test types. Available at: https://www.fda.gov/news-events/press-announcements/coronavirus-covid-19-update-fda-updates-covid-19-test-policy-encourages-developers-seek-traditional. Accessed 10/5/2022.
19. Fact sheet: the Biden administration announces Americans can order additional free at-home. Rapid COVID-19 Tests at COVIDTests.gov Available at: https://www.whitehouse.gov/briefing-room/statements-releases/2022/05/17/fact-sheet-the-biden-administration-announces-americans-can-order-additional-free-at-home-rapid-covid-19-tests-at-covidtests-gov/. Accessed 10/5/2022.
20. Clinical laboratory improvement advisory committee (CLIAC), April 2022, Sheldon Campbell. Current and future applications of point-of-care testing – the laboratory perspective. Available at: https://www.cdc.gov/cliac/past-meetings.html. Accessed 10/7/2022.
21. Available at: https://www.ondemand.labcorp.com/blog/why-confirming-rapid-antigen-covid-19-test-results-pcr-testimoportant#:~:text=Given%20rapid%20tests%20lower%20sensivitities,as%20a%20%E2%80%9Csecond%20opinion%E2%80%9D. Accessed November 19, 2022.
22. Cordero P, Weiss M, Trinh C, et al A comparison of viral culture, DFA and xTag RVP assays for the detection of respiratory viral agents during the H1N1 pandemic. Clinical Virology Symposium Daytona Beach, Fla April 25-28, 2010.
23. Irwin Z. Rothenberg. Strategies necessary to achieve quality waived testing. Available at: https://www.physiciansofficeresource.com/articles/point-of-care-testing/quality-waived-testing/. Accessed 10/16/2022.
24. Ginocchio CC, Zhang F, Manji R, et al. Evaluation of multiple test methods for the detection of the novel 2009 influenza A (H1N1) during the New York City outbreak. J Clin Virol 2009;45(3):191–5.
25. How flu viruses can change: "drift" and "shift". Available at: https://www.cdc.gov/flu/about/viruses/change.htm. Accessed Oct 15, 2022.
26. SARS-CoV-2 viral mutations: impact on COVID-19 tests. Available at: https://www.fda.gov/medical-devices/coronavirus-covid-19-and-medical-devices/sars-cov-2-viral-mutations-impact-covid-19-tests. Accessed 10/15/2022.
27. 2009 H1N1 pandemic timeline. Available at: https://www.cdc.gov/flu/pandemic-resources/2009-pandemic-timeline.html. Accessed 10/9/2022.
28. National COVID-19 preparedness plan. Available at: https://www.whitehouse.gov/covidplan/. Accessed 10/16/2022.
29. Halstead DC, Sautter RL. A literature review on how we can address medical laboratory scientist staffing shortages. Lab Med 2022;lmac090. https://doi.org/10.1093/labmed/lmac090, published online ahead of print, 2022 Sep 23.

Practical Challenges of Point-of-Care Testing

Daniel A. Ortiz, PhD, D(ABMM)ᵃ, Michael J. Loeffelholz, PhD, D(ABMM)ᵇ,*

KEYWORDS

- Point-of-care testing • POCT • Quality • Performance

KEY POINTS

- The costs of rapid point-of-care testing (POCT) need to be weighed against the clinical benefit and operational impact to determine if POCT is appropriate based on the practical challenges at each institution.
- The practical challenges of point-of-care testing (POCT) include analytical performance and quality compared with testing performed in a central laboratory as well as higher cost per test compared to more automated, laboratory-based tests.
- These challenges can be addressed with new test technology, instituting a quality management system and data connectivity in the POCT setting, consensus and practice guidelines for the use of POCT, and studies that demonstrate clinical and economic value of POCT.

INTRODUCTION

Point-of-care testing (POCT) refers to diagnostic tests performed at or near the site of a patient rather than in a traditional laboratory setting. POCT results are rapid and can provide actionable information that leads to changes in patient management. Rapid results for infectious disease testing improve patient care by reducing the need for multiple patient visits, facilitating appropriate and timely treatment, and preventing further spread of disease.[1–4] Along with these POCT benefits come many practical challenges that need to be considered both before implementing as well as performing POCT. There is limited value in POCT if rapid results will not change patient management. The lack of algorithms and guidelines incorporating POCT into infectious disease diagnoses can deter providers from implementing POCT. In addition, health care providers may have little confidence in POCT results due to real or perceived concerns with diagnostic accuracy compared with laboratory-based testing.[5–8] Although point-of-care (POC) lateral flow antigen and antibody tests tend to have lower

ᵃ Microbiology and Molecular Pathology, Department of Pathology, Oakland University William Beaumont School of Medicine, Beaumont Health, 3601 West 13 Mile Road, Royal Oak, MI 48073, USA; ᵇ Scientific Affairs, Cepheid, 1324 Chesapeake Terrace, Sunnyvale, CA 94089, USA
* Corresponding author.
E-mail address: Michael.loeffelholz@cepheid.com

Clin Lab Med 43 (2023) 155–165
https://doi.org/10.1016/j.cll.2023.02.002
0272-2712/23/© 2023 Elsevier Inc. All rights reserved.

labmed.theclinics.com

sensitivity, they still have clinical utility if used in the appropriate setting.[9–11] Also, some molecular POC tests have demonstrated similar performance characteristics to laboratory-based tests.[11–14] The tradeoff between POCT and laboratory-based testing should be discussed with health care providers to determine if POCT results will have a significant impact on patient management decisions such as prescribing antivirals/antibiotics, ordering additional tests, or triaging patients.

Because the clinical benefit of POCT depends on the rapid time to result, POCT sites should strive to make results available during the patient encounter. This can be challenging depending on the daily workload, patient care workflow, and POCT device. Adding POCT responsibilities to an already busy workforce may not always be feasible, and additional staff may be needed to perform POCT, especially if high test volumes are anticipated. Patient care workflows may also have to be adjusted based on the hands-on time, turnaround time, and throughput of the POCT device. Ideally, POCT should integrate seamlessly with the daily workflow and provide results in a timely manner.

The clinical benefit of a rapid result may be outweighed by the overall cost of POCT. The price per test will increase compared with laboratory-based tests due to POCT reagents being manufactured as single-use tests. If instrumentation is required, additional expenses will be incurred by the POCT site for capital equipment purchases and service contracts. There are also many hidden POCT costs associated with training, quality control, quality assurance, proficiency testing, connectivity, and data management. To justify the additional expense of POCT, a cost-benefit analysis should be conducted, taking into account improvements in clinical and operational outcomes.

Although infectious disease POCT is an attractive option, it may not always be beneficial or feasible to implement. Difficulties in measuring the clinical benefit and operational impact, as well as cost are just a few of the challenges associated with POCT. There are many other factors to consider (location, staff, test performance, and so on) that may be barriers to implementing and performing POCT. Identifying the practical challenges associated with POCT can help facilities determine if POCT is appropriate for their location or patient population. In a systematic review of the literature, the most prevalent barriers to adoption of POCT included economics of adoption (costs) and concerns about quality assurance (including untrained users)[6] (**Table 1**).

CLINICAL APPLICATION

The main goal of POCT is to replace or augment traditional laboratory testing with a rapid, clinically actionable result that will improve patient care and outcomes. However, concerns about the reduced analytical accuracy or performance of POCT compared with laboratory-based tests are a significant barrier to the adoption of POCT. With the POCT landscape constantly evolving, it can be challenging for health care providers to remain up to date and understand the nuances and performance of each test method, device, and disease. Although test manufacturers provide test performance data from clinical trials in their device package inserts, independent studies that provide real world performance data are important to support package insert claims and demonstrate clinical utility in a POC setting.

POINT-OF-CARE TESTING VERSUS CENTRAL LABORATORY TESTS

As previously mentioned, one of the main barriers to POCT implementation is the reduced analytical performance of some POC tests compared with methods performed in the laboratory.[6] POC tests often have lower diagnostic sensitivity than laboratory-based tests due to reduced analytical sensitivity associated with inherent assay design features such as the absence of a target amplification step or abbreviated

Table 1
Point-of-care testing—challenges and solutions

Characteristic	Challenges	Solutions
Guidelines, including POCT algorithms	• Absent • Lack of consensus	• Development of practice guidelines that incorporate POCT
Accuracy of POCT	• POCT may have reduced analytical performance compared with laboratory-based tests • Test device operation by untrained users	• Technology, including nucleic acid amplification • Instrument-read POCT devices • Comprehensive training and ongoing competency assessments
Cost compared with laboratory-based tests	• POC tests may have higher reagent costs per test than laboratory-based tests	• Factor institutional cost savings often provided by POCT
Staff and clinic workflow	• Incorporating POCT into daily workflow • Additional staff responsibilities • Testing volumes	• Appropriate POC test device selection • Instrumentation and connectivity • Additional staffing
Quality	• Reduced quality, often associated with untrained users • Data management and compliance with regulatory requirements	• Comprehensive training and ongoing competency assessments • Institute POCT quality management system led by a laboratory medicine professional • Input POCT results to the electronic medical record • Use bidirectional communication of POC instruments

amplification, manually read lateral flow immunoassay, or antigen detection. The lower limit of detection of rapid antigen tests can be several logs higher than that of real-time polymerase chain reaction (RT-PCR).[15,16] For example, SARS-CoV-2 antigen tests will generally be positive in specimens with RT-PCR cycle threshold values of 30 and lower,[17,18] resulting in average diagnostic sensitivity ranging from approximately 29% to 98% depending on the patient population.[19] The specificity of rapid antigen tests is usually high.[10,19,20] Before the Food and Drug Administration reclassification of influenza rapid antigen tests to class II devices and requiring at least 80% sensitivity, these tests often had sensitivities ranging from approximately 50% to 60% compared with RT-PCR.[20] Some POC nucleic acid amplification tests (NAATs) have reduced sensitivity compared with laboratory-based NAATs due to their abbreviated amplification step in order to shorten the time to result.[21,22] This compromise in sensitivity is not universal among POC NAATs, with some demonstrating equivalent performance to laboratory-based NAATs.[11–14,23] Although the accuracy of POCT is often compared with central laboratory tests, POCT sites should place greater emphasis on the clinical benefit rather than the diagnostic accuracy to determine if POCT is appropriate. Infectious disease POCT can provide better linkage to care with less follow-up visits and more appropriate use of antibiotics and antivirals.

Instrumentation

The most common infectious disease POCT devices are manual, handheld lateral flow immunoassays that detect specific proteins (antigens) of the pathogen. These visually read lateral flow immunoassays have an inherent limit to analytical sensitivity due to operator subjectivity and expertise. An instrument-read POCT device increases the diagnostic accuracy by removing operator bias and improving the limit of detection. In fact, fluorescent immunoassays that detect influenza virus antigen have been shown to be significantly more sensitive than manually read, colorimetric immunoassays.[24,25] Instrument-read POC tests also ensure the operator is following the manufacturer's instructions and product labeling. Some instrument design features can even eliminate or reduce the risk of errors such as the use of expired reagents, quality control frequency, improper analytical steps (eg, incubation time), and incorrect documentation.[26] Instrumentation combined with connectivity to a hospital or laboratory information system can also help expedite patient results and prevent the release of inaccurate results.

Point-of-Care Testing Guidelines

Infectious disease guidelines and recommendations are main drivers of the clinical decision process. Although some POCT guidelines exist (eg, hepatitis C virus, human immunodeficiency virus [HIV]),[27,28] others lack clearly defined indications for POCT in an outpatient setting, which makes it challenging to determine the clinical need. For example, outpatient POCT guidelines for influenza are often vague and provide limited diagnosis and treatment decisions.[29,30] With the recent advances in POCT, the development of new guidelines often falls behind.

Even when guidelines or recommendations are available, there can be a lack of consensus on how to use POCT for diagnosis and treatment. An example is group A *Streptococcus* (GAS), where a Bayesian scoring system based on clinical symptoms is used to predict the probability of streptococcal infection and when to perform a rapid antigen detection test (RADT). Some guidelines recommend against performing an RADT and empirically treating patients with a score greater than or equal to 4, whereas others recommend always performing an RADT because clinical features are unreliable in differentiating between GAS and viral pharyngitis.[31,32] Standardization among the different groups is needed to provide clear and concise guidelines for incorporating POCT into clinical practice.

Determining the clinical need may depend on internal evaluation studies of the POCT site. Each POC site should consider evaluating POC test performance against laboratory-based tests and define acceptable performance standards; this may be POCT device dependent, as the Cochrane review of GAS pharyngitis in children states that "Whether negative RADTs should be backed up by throat culture depends mainly on the reported sensitivity of the test."[10] On the other hand, European guidelines have dropped the requirement for reflex cultures in pediatric populations altogether when the RADT is negative.[33] Ultimately, the clinical need may depend on performance characteristics, location, and patient population of the POCT site.

ECONOMICS OF POINT-OF-CARE TESTING ADOPTION

A simple cost analysis of POCT will often yield a higher cost per test compared with laboratory-based testing and can be a major issue in the justification of its adoption. Direct costs of POCT may include the purchase of instruments along with consumables such as disposable test cartridges and reagents, whereas indirect costs relate to staffing, training, quality control, quality assurance, proficiency testing, connectivity, and data management. However, POCT does provide quicker time to result, which can lead to quicker treatment, reduced visits and downstream laboratory costs, and overall increased patient satisfaction.[1–4] The challenge is quantifying the clinical and operational benefit to justify the higher cost per test, especially when the laboratory testing budget and clinical budget are seen as two separate entities. Viewing the institution as a whole can help realize potential savings across the organization by including anticipated cost savings from better use of resources (eg, less patient transfers to an acute area hospital) and patient outcomes (eg, morbidity and mortality) in the cost-benefit analysis. With limited outcome data available from POCT in the primary care setting, a multidisciplinary approach from various stake holders is necessary to provide cost justification data.

POINT-OF-CARE TESTING LOCATION

Infectious disease POCT devices are often small and portable, which allows them to be used in a variety of settings, including emergency departments, skilled nursing facilities, long-term care facilities, nursing homes, physician offices, and pharmacies. However, POCT sites need to be evaluated to determine if the facility is appropriately equipped to conduct POCT. The specimen type, test volume, and test device can change the POCT site requirements.

The evaluation of the specimen collection space should take into account the specimen type needed for testing. Specimen types with low risk of potential exposure (eg, whole blood, serum, or plasma) can be conducted safely indoors with limited protection barriers. Other specimen types, such as throat or nasopharyngeal swabs, have a higher risk of potential exposure due to the patient coughing or sneezing during the collection process. High-risk specimen types should be collected with additional personal protective equipment, and patient collection sites should be separated by distance or physical barriers (eg, individual rooms or privacy curtains). Outdoor or drive-through collection sites can also be used to mitigate risks of potential exposure to health care personnel and other patients.

Once the specimen is collected, testing can occur in the same room as the patient or an adjacent room or space. The location of the testing site will depend on the test device and the infrastructure of the facility. The test device or instrumentation may require additional safety precautions if aerosols are at risk of being produced such as a biosafety cabinet, splash guard, or face shield. Testing locations should have ample space to perform testing and may require centrifuges for processing serum or plasma samples, electrical or data connection ports, and refrigerators for specimen or regent storage. POCT devices also have temperature and humidity requirements that must be followed to ensure accurate test performance[34,35]; this is especially important for testing performed in the field or a mobile setting where temperature and humidity can be difficult to control. Although POCT has made infectious disease testing more accessible, the collection and testing location are important factors to consider before implementation.

STAFFING

Implementing POCT can have a significant impact on the workload of health care staff. The primary role of health care providers is taking care of the patient, and adding additional POCT responsibilities may compromise patient care. Current staffing shortages in the health care industry can also be a significant barrier to implementation. It is important to account for staffing beyond the need for performing POCT. Staff is also needed for training, inventory management, equipment maintenance, quality assurance, and regulatory compliance.

POCT staff also consist of nonlaboratory personnel with varying levels of education and experience (eg, pharmacists, nurses, medical assistants). They are often unfamiliar with routine laboratory practices and preanalytical, analytical, and postanalytical variables that can affect POCT results. Staff need to be educated and trained on proper specimen collection, storage (if applicable), and testing to be compliant with CLIA regulations and ensure accurate test results. This initial training should be followed by competency assessments at specific intervals to maintain staff proficiency and minimize potential errors. For instance, Fox and colleagues found differences between laboratory technologists and nontechnical personnel when performing a rapid GAS antigen test that required a manual read for interpretation. Test sensitivity was consistently greater when the test was performed by laboratory technologists than when it was performed by nonlaboratory personnel (*P* < .0001).[36] This difference in test sensitivity was attributed to the lack of operator experience and feedback, which can be improved through regular competency or proficiency testing.

QUALITY

One of the most frequently cited barriers to the adoption of POCT is concern of poor quality, usually associated with untrained users.[6] Implementation of a quality management system helps to ensure high quality in the POC setting.[37] There are several sources for POCT quality guidelines and standards, including the College of American Pathologists (CAP) and The Joint Commission. The Clinical and Laboratory Standards Institute (CLSI) has published several guidelines on POCT quality, including POCT07, *"Quality management: Approaches to Reducing Errors at the Point of Care; Approved Guideline,"* and POCT08, *"Quality Practices in Noninstrumented Point-of-Care Testing: an Instructional Manual and Resources for Healthcare Workers; Approved Guideline."*

PREANALYTICAL AND ANALYTICAL FACTORS

Although POCT devices are relatively simple and easy to perform, errors can occur at any point throughout the testing process. The accuracy of any POC test heavily depends on appropriate specimen collection. Potential errors in collection that could lead to erroneous test results include squeezing too hard for capillary samples, inadequate filling of collection devices, or sampling the wrong anatomic site. The timing of specimen collection may also be important. For instance, acute HIV or syphilis infections may not be detected if testing is performed at early stages of infection.[38–41] In contrast, respiratory infections may not be detected at later stages of infection because test sensitivity declines the further out from symptom onset. False-positive results are also more likely to occur if testing is performed when disease prevalence is low (eg, testing for influenza during the summer months).[42,43] In some of these situations, laboratory-based testing is preferred over POCT, and facilities should clearly define when specimens should be sent to a reference laboratory for analysis. Because of their high analytical sensitivity, NAATs are at greater risk for environmental contamination than rapid antigen tests. Careful attention to the manufacturer's instructions is important to prevent environmental contamination, and this depends on the setting in which the tests are performed and the skill level of the test operators. It is important to understand the risk of environmental contamination of NAATs in the actual setting in which they will be used such as the POC setting.[44]

In a POC setting, the same health care provider often performs specimen collection, processing, and testing to reduce the risk of preanalytical errors. However, this workflow may not be feasible for all POCT sites, and specimens may need to be stored before testing or tested by another health care provider. If specimens are stored before testing, the manufacturer's storage requirements must be followed to prevent specimen degradation that can lead to false-negative results.[45] After storage or specimen transfer, POCT personnel should reverify the patient identity (ie, 2 patient identifiers) and test being performed. Specimens without appropriate identifiers should not be tested to avoid inaccurate reporting of results that could cause patient harm. Facilities using a manual or paper process are more prone to specimen labeling errors and should consider an electronic ordering system that automatically generates patient labels with each test order. POCT instruments with barcode readers and electronic medical record (EMR) interfacing capabilities can further reduce the chance of inaccurate reporting, but these features often come with additional costs. Identifying the appropriate workflow to minimize preanalytical errors will be institution and POCT device dependent.

The type of POCT device used can also introduce additional risks of analytical errors occurring during the testing process. POCT devices may come with instrumentation that has specific requirements for daily, monthly, or designated maintenance. Adherence to this maintenance program is essential for quality POCT results and should also be performed after significant events that could affect instrument performance, such as physically moving the instrument, or when test or quality control results indicate nonconformance. Errors can also occur if the manufacturers' storage instructions (eg, room temperature or refrigerated) are not followed. If refrigeration is required, POCT kits and reagents must be allowed to come to room temperature before testing. Neglecting appropriate storage or testing conditions can reduce test accuracy. Test accuracy also depends on the level of experience of the user, especially when a manual read is required. Although the need for a manual read is circumvented by the use of an automated reader, many antigen-based POCT devices still require a manual read. This emphasizes the importance of a robust training program for POCT staff to minimize analytical errors and ensure accurate results.

POSTANALYTICAL FACTORS (REPORTING OF POINT-OF-CARE TESTING RESULTS)

A barrier to the adoption of POCT is the challenge of data connectivity and resulting data management.[6] The variety of POCT instruments, devices, testing personnel, and locations makes the data management challenging. Many POC tests are noninstrumented, such as lateral flow devices; this requires manual entry of device and user information and test results into a hospital management system. POCT results should be added to the EMR to allow monitoring of test and quality control results but separately from laboratory test results for quality assurance purposes.[46] The CLSI has published a standard POCT01, *"Point-of-Care Connectivity Approved Standard—Second Edition,"* which provides context for bidirectional communication of POC instruments.

IMPLEMENTING A QUALITY MANAGEMENT SYSTEM

Execution of a quality management system, including testing of quality control materials at a regular frequency, and participation in proficiency testing or external quality assessment (EQA) programs will improve the quality of POCT results.[37] Most molecular POC tests incorporate control material within the test device (internal control), and this can be monitored (rate of invalid test results) similar to the results of external quality control and EQA. Some molecular tests incorporate an additional control for specimen adequacy or quality. This type of control specifically amplifies and detects an ubiquitous human gene (often a housekeeping gene) present in all cells.[47] A negative specimen adequacy control result will invalidate the test and can be caused by failure to add specimen to the collection device (or to the test device), an insufficiently collected specimen, inhibitory substances in the specimen, or test device failure. Quality metrics can be another element of a quality management system. Quality metrics are measurements of test data and then evaluating those data over time to monitor the test process. Examples of POCT quality metrics include external quality control results, internal (built-in) quality control if present in a test, test positivity rates, and error or invalid rates. Trending quality metrics data can detect defects in test devices, nonconformance to testing protocols, or contamination. In order to achieve the greatest benefit, these quality management programs should be supported by a professional clinical laboratory scientist.[37] Health care systems and integrated delivery networks, consisting of both a core laboratory medically directed by pathologists or doctoral-level clinical laboratory scientists, as well as POCT, have the ability to designate a laboratory medicine professional to oversee the POCT quality management system.

SUMMARY

The infectious disease POCT landscape is constantly improving but many of the practical challenges of implementing POCT still remain. With the wide variety of testing options available, many organizations struggle with choosing the appropriate POCT device due to limited/absent guidelines or acceptable accuracy levels when compared with laboratory-based tests. Even with the improved diagnostic accuracy of molecular POC tests, the financial impact of implementing POCT continues to be problematic. Data on the impact and cost-effectiveness of POCT are complex and difficult to gauge in the primary care setting. More evidence-based clinical and economic benefit studies are needed to support use of rapid results in a POC setting. Ultimately, the decision to implement POCT is institution dependent and will differ based on the practical challenges associated with POCT at their location.

CLINICS CARE POINTS

- A clinical and operational needs assessment can determine the impact of POCT on patient management and clinical care pathways.
- The additional expense of POCT can be justified by moving away from the traditional "siloed budgeting" approach and considering cost savings to the entire organization.
- Newer POCT technology and connectivity can improve diagnostic accuracy and quality assurance.
- Implementation of a quality management system helps to ensure that POCT results are accurate and reliable.

DISCLOSURE

M.J. Loeffelholz receives salary from Cepheid; D.A. Ortiz is a paid scientific advisor for Beckman Coulter, Quidel, and MiraVista.

REFERENCES

1. Teoh TK, Powell J, Kelly J, et al. Outcomes of point-of-care testing for influenza in the emergency department of a tertiary referral hospital in Ireland. J Hosp Infect 2021;110:45–51.

2. Rönn MM, Menzies NA, Gift TL, et al. Potential for point-of-care tests to reduce Chlamydia-associated Burden in the United States: a Mathematical Modeling analysis. Clin Infect Dis 2020;70(9):1816–23.

3. Benirschke RC, McElvania E, Thomson RB, et al. Clinical impact of rapid point-of-care PCR influenza testing in an Urgent care setting: a single-center study. J Clin Microbiol 2019;57(3).

4. Rao A, Berg B, Quezada T, et al. Diagnosis and antibiotic treatment of group a streptococcal pharyngitis in children in a primary care setting: impact of point-of-care polymerase chain reaction. BMC Pediatr 2019;19(1):24.

5. Pai NP, Wilkinson S, Deli-Houssein R, et al. Barriers to implementation of rapid and point-of-care tests for human Immunodeficiency virus infection: Findings from a systematic review (1996-2014). Point Care 2015;14(3):81–7.

6. Quinn AD, Dixon D, Meenan BJ. Barriers to hospital-based clinical adoption of point-of-care testing (POCT): a systematic narrative review. Crit Rev Clin Lab Sci 2016;53(1):1–12.

7. Hocking L, George J, Broberg EK, et al. Point of care testing for infectious disease in europe: a scoping review and survey study. Front Public Health 2021; 9:722943.

8. Hardy V, Thompson M, Alto W, et al. Exploring the barriers and facilitators to use of point of care tests in family medicine clinics in the United States. BMC Fam Pract 2016;17(1):149.

9. Meggi B, Bollinger T, Mabunda N, et al. Point-of-care p24 infant testing for HIV may increase patient Identification despite low sensitivity. PLoS One 2017; 12(1):e0169497.

10. Cohen JF, Bertille N, Cohen R, et al. Rapid antigen detection test for group A streptococcus in children with pharyngitis. Cochrane Database Syst Rev 2016; 7:CD010502.

11. Merckx J, Wali R, Schiller I, et al. Diagnostic accuracy of Novel and traditional rapid tests for influenza infection compared with Reverse Transcriptase polymerase chain reaction: a systematic review and meta-analysis. Ann Intern Med 2017; 167(6):394–409.

12. Banerjee D, Kanwar N, Hassan F, et al. Comparison of Six Sample-to-Answer influenza A/B and respiratory Syncytial virus nucleic acid amplification assays using respiratory specimens from children. J Clin Microbiol 2018;56(11). https://doi.org/10.1128/JCM.00930-18.

13. Hansen G, Marino J, Wang Z-X, et al. Clinical performance of the point-of-care cobas Liat for detection of SARS-CoV-2 in 20 Minutes: a Multicenter study. J Clin Microbiol 2021;59(2). https://doi.org/10.1128/JCM.02811-20.

14. Wolters F, van de Bovenkamp J, van den Bosch B, et al. Multi-center evaluation of cepheid xpert® xpress SARS-CoV-2 point-of-care test during the SARS-CoV-2 pandemic. J Clin Virol 2020;128:104426.

15. Mak GC, Lau SS, Wong KK, et al. Analytical sensitivity and clinical sensitivity of the three rapid antigen detection kits for detection of SARS-CoV-2 virus. J Clin Virol 2020;133:104684.

16. Chan KH, Chan KM, Ho YL, et al. Quantitative analysis of four rapid antigen assays for detection of pandemic H1N1 2009 compared with seasonal H1N1 and H3N2 influenza A viruses on nasopharyngeal aspirates from patients with influenza. J Virol Methods 2012;186(1–2):184–8.

17. Young S, Taylor SN, Cammarata CL, et al. Clinical evaluation of BD Veritor SARS-CoV-2 point-of-care test performance compared to PCR-based testing and

versus the Sofia 2 SARS antigen point-of-care test. J Clin Microbiol 2020;59(1). https://doi.org/10.1128/JCM.02338-20.

18. Osterman A, Badell I, Basara E, et al. Impaired detection of omicron by SARS-CoV-2 rapid antigen tests. Med Microbiol Immunol 2022;211(2–3):105–17. https://doi.org/10.1007/s00430-022-00730-z.

19. Hayer J, Kasapic D, Zemmrich C. Real-world clinical performance of commercial SARS-CoV-2 rapid antigen tests in suspected COVID-19: a systematic meta-analysis of available data as of November 20, 2020. Int J Infect Dis 2021;108: 592–602.

20. Peaper DR, Landry ML. Rapid diagnosis of influenza: state of the art. Clin Lab Med 2014;34(2):365–85.

21. Zhen W, Smith E, Manji R, et al. Clinical evaluation of three Sample-to-Answer Platforms for detection of SARS-CoV-2. J Clin Microbiol 2020;58(8). https://doi.org/10.1128/JCM.00783-20.

22. Hogan CA, Garamani N, Lee AS, et al. Comparison of the Accula SARS-CoV-2 test with a laboratory-Developed assay for detection of SARS-CoV-2 RNA in clinical nasopharyngeal specimens. J Clin Microbiol 2020;58(8). https://doi.org/10.1128/JCM.01072-20.

23. Moran A, Beavis KG, Matushek SM, et al. Detection of SARS-CoV-2 by Use of the cepheid xpert xpress SARS-CoV-2 and Roche cobas SARS-CoV-2 assays. J Clin Microbiol 2020;58(8). https://doi.org/10.1128/JCM.00772-20.

24. Calabria D, Calabretta MM, Zangheri M, et al. Recent Advancements in Enzyme-based lateral flow immunoassays. Sensors (Basel) 2021;21(10). https://doi.org/10.3390/s21103358.

25. Lee CK, Cho CH, Woo MK, et al. Evaluation of Sofia fluorescent immunoassay analyzer for influenza A/B virus. J Clin Virol 2012;55(3):239–43.

26. Lewandrowski K, Gregory K, Macmillan D. Assuring quality in point-of-care testing: evolution of technologies, informatics, and program management. Arch Pathol Lab Med 2011;135(11):1405–14.

27. HCV testing and linkage to care | HCV guidance. Available at: https://www.hcvguidelines.org/evaluate/testing-and-linkage. Accessed December 22, 2022.

28. Prenatal and Perinatal human Immunodeficiency virus testing | ACOG. Available at: https://www.acog.org/clinical/clinical-guidance/committee-opinion/articles/2018/09/prenatal-and-perinatal-human-immunodeficiency-virus-testing. Accessed December 22, 2022.

29. Guidelines for the clinical management of severe illness from influenza virus infections. Geneva: World Health Organization; 2022.

30. Uyeki TM, Bernstein HH, Bradley JS, et al. Clinical practice guidelines by the infectious diseases society of America: 2018 update on diagnosis, treatment, chemoprophylaxis, and institutional outbreak management of seasonal influenzaa. Clin Infect Dis 2019;68(6):e1–47.

31. Shulman ST, Bisno AL, Clegg HW, et al. Clinical practice guideline for the diagnosis and management of group A streptococcal pharyngitis: 2012 update by the Infectious Diseases Society of America. Clin Infect Dis 2012;55(10):e86–102.

32. Sauve L, Forrester AM, Top KA. Group A streptococcal pharyngitis: a practical guide to diagnosis and treatment. Paediatr Child Health 2021;26(5):319–20.

33. ESCMID Sore Throat Guideline Group, Pelucchi C, Grigoryan L, et al. Guideline for the management of acute sore throat. Clin Microbiol Infect 2012;18(Suppl 1):1–28.

34. Pollock NR, Jacobs JR, Tran K, et al. Performance and implementation evaluation of the Abbott BinaxNOW rapid antigen test in a high-throughput drive-through

community testing site in Massachusetts. J Clin Microbiol 2021;59(5). https://doi.org/10.1128/JCM.00083-21.

35. Bienek DR, Charlton DG. The effect of simulated field storage conditions on the accuracy of rapid user-friendly blood pathogen detection kits. Mil Med 2012; 177(5):583–8.

36. Fox JW, Cohen DM, Marcon MJ, et al. Performance of rapid streptococcal antigen testing varies by personnel. J Clin Microbiol 2006;44(11):3918–22.

37. Price CP, Smith I, Van den Bruel A. Improving the quality of point-of-care testing. Fam Pract 2018;35(4):358–64.

38. Angel-Müller E, Grillo-Ardila CF, Amaya-Guio J, et al. Point of care rapid test for diagnosis of syphilis infection in men and nonpregnant women. Cochrane Database Syst Rev May 2018. https://doi.org/10.1002/14651858.CD013036.

39. Rosenberg NE, Kamanga G, Phiri S, et al. Detection of acute HIV infection: a field evaluation of the determine® HIV-1/2 Ag/Ab combo test. J Infect Dis 2012;205(4): 528–34.

40. Conway DP, Holt M, McNulty A, et al. Multi-centre evaluation of the Determine HIV Combo assay when used for point of care testing in a high risk clinic-based population. PLoS One 2014;9(4):e94062.

41. Duong YT, Mavengere Y, Patel H, et al. Poor performance of the determine HIV-1/2 Ag/Ab combo fourth-generation rapid test for detection of acute infections in a National Household Survey in Swaziland. J Clin Microbiol 2014;52(10):3743–8.

42. Mutnal MB, Lanham JA, Walker K, et al. False positive Influenza rapid tests using newly EUA cleared multiplex assay in a low prevalence setting. J Med Virol 2021; 93(6):3285.

43. Skittrall JP, Wilson M, Smielewska AA, et al. Specificity and positive predictive value of SARS-CoV-2 nucleic acid amplification testing in a low-prevalence setting. Clin Microbiol Infect 2021;27(3). 469.e9-469.e15.

44. Donato LJ, Myhre NK, Murray MA, et al. Assessment of test performance and potential for environmental contamination associated with a point-of-care molecular assay for group A Streptococcus in an End user setting. J Clin Microbiol 2019; 57(2). https://doi.org/10.1128/JCM.01629-18.

45. Kelly K. Pre-analytical errors in rapid influenza testing. Clin Infect Dis 2010;50(6): 935, author reply 936-7.

46. Fung AWS. Utilizing connectivity and data management system for effective quality management and regulatory compliance in point of care testing. Pract Lab Med 2020;22:e00187.

47. Deviaene M, Weigel KM, Wood RC, et al. Sample adequacy controls for infectious disease diagnosis by oral swabbing. PLoS One 2020;15(10):e0241542.

Will Antigen Testing Remain Relevant in the Point-of-Care Testing Environment?

Lindsey E. Nielsen, PhD, D(ABMM)[a,*], Steven Mahlen, PhD, D(ABMM)[b], Deena E. Sutter, MD[c]

KEYWORDS

- Antigen assay • Point-of-care • Waived testing • Molecular assay
- Pathogen detection • Diagnostic infectious diease assay

KEY POINTS

- Molecular testing platforms typically provide optimal sensitivity and specificity for detection of infectious pathogens.
- Historical barriers to implementing molecular assays include cost-per-test, reimbursement rate, need for a higher level of staff training, and specific requirements for infrastructure.
- Multianalyte molecular testing reduces the total number of assays performed and reduces the time to diagnosis with a significant advantage over older molecular assays.
- Many antigen platforms require negative results to be reflexed to a molecular assay for confirmation, with resultant increased costs and delays in diagnosis.
- Overcoming barriers to implementation and costs associated with molecular platforms may enable point-of-care laboratories to eliminate most antigenic assays in favor of more sensitive and accurate nucleic acid testing platforms.

INTRODUCTION AND BACKGROUND

Before the molecular age, cell culture was the gold standard for confirmatory diagnosis of viral and atypical infectious diseases. Typical cell culture methodologies are costly, require days (or weeks) for results, and require significant technical expertise. As a result, cell culture is impractical for timely diagnostic testing in most of the health care environments, especially in point-of-care (POC) testing environments. Traditional bacterial culture methods, although typically less complex than cell culture, also have disadvantages due to the need for incubation, subsequent identification of pathogens, and significant technical expertise.

[a] LN Laboratory Consulting, NE, USA; [b] Sanford Health, Bismark, ND, USA; [c] Tenet Physician Resources/Baptist Health System, San Antonio, TX, USA
* Corresponding author. LN Laboratory Consulting, LLC, Wood River, NE, USA.
E-mail address: lindseynielsenpc@gmail.com

Clin Lab Med 43 (2023) 167–179
https://doi.org/10.1016/j.cll.2023.02.003
0272-2712/23/© 2023 Elsevier Inc. All rights reserved.
labmed.theclinics.com

The introduction of antigen diagnostic tests that detect protein of a pathogen revolutionized the POC setting. The ease of sample collection, specimen manipulation, and test performance in the POC environment has made antigen testing a common practice in multiple settings, from provider offices to hospital laboratories. In context of ideal diagnostic tests, antigen assays fulfilled many of the World Health Organization ASSURED criteria relative to culture or preexisting diagnostic methods, that is, they are affordable, sensitive, specific, user-friendly, rapid/robust, equipment-free, and deliverable.[1–3]

Another option for diagnostic testing is molecular assays, often referred to as nucleic acid amplification tests (NAATs). These options provide several advantages over antigen testing based on reliability but were not routinely available in the POC setting based on meeting the ASSURED criteria. Molecular assays increasingly meet ASSURED criteria and are being used as replacements for antigen-based assays due to technology advances and elimination of cumbersome, multistep processing protocols. Other health care system advances, such as use of computerized electronic health records (EHR) and laboratory information system (LIS), have allowed for interfacing of NAAT results and alleviated the requirement for manual transcription of antigen results. The use of computerized systems and considerations for specimen collections have prompted WHO to update the ASSURED criteria to RE-ASSURED, which includes real-time connectivity and ease of specimen collection.[2,4]

One advantage that more sensitive molecular systems have over antigen assays is a reduced requirement for confirmatory testing of negative results, leading to increased confidence in accuracy of results. Still, multiple obstacles remain for NAATs to be widely accepted and used in the POC setting. Barriers such as cost of processing, POC infrastructure and design, and increased need for staff training and expertise may delay implementation of NAAT tests. This article discusses the general considerations of antigen and molecular assays and the merits and factors to consider when implementing diagnostic assays for several common pathogens.

General Considerations

When selecting a platform for diagnostic assays universal considerations include the test performance, need for confirmation, time-to-diagnosis, risk of false results and impact on public health, limit of detection, laboratory infrastructure, and cost and reimbursement rates.5

Assay Performance

Molecular assays will often have higher sensitivities than antigen assays[6–9]; this is directly related to the limit of detection of the NAAT method that can accurately detect very low quantities of the pathogen's nucleic acid. NAAT assays detect as few as 10 to 100 copies of the targeted nucleic acid sequence. The amplification of a targeted gene or genetic marker, coupled with sensitive detection methods such as fluorescence, allows detection of the pathogen's signature (analyte) at earlier stages of infection or disease and well before the concentration of any antigen allows detection via antigen assays. Hence, the limit of detection of a molecular assay is always much lower than with any antigenic method.[10]

A diagnostic assay's performance is generally measured by its sensitivity and specificity as compared with an established "gold standard." The gold standard was traditionally culture-based, but in the modern era, the baseline comparator is more often a molecular assay. Relatively high-sensitivity and -specificity assays may have widely variable positive and negative predictive values depending on disease incidence and prevalence; this concept is critically important to relay to clinicians for appropriate interpretation of results. In general, antigen-based tests will have a better predictive value during periods of higher disease prevalence than low prevalence despite their lower sensitivity than NAAT assays. There is typically less variation in negative and positive predictive values using molecular methods because the sensitivity and specificity of NAATs are superior to antigen assays. Thus, antigen assays generally perform less optimally when a pathogen is associated with dynamic seasonal variations.

Specificity between molecular and antigen-based testing methods are generally comparable for overall diagnostic purposes. The specificity for influenza A and B, for example, is greater than 98% for both molecular and most antigen methods and provides an accurate diagnosis for a positive test result. Group A *Streptococcus* (GAS), *Trichomonas*, and SARS-CoV-2 are additional examples of similar specificity between antigen and NAAT performance, whereas other antigen tests are lower (**Table 1**).

Assay Confirmation

Most antigen assays suggest confirmatory testing by molecular methods due to relatively low limit-of-detection, sensitivity, and, occasionally, specificity. It is important to understand the need for confirmatory testing, as, in the case of a negative antigen result, there are 2 possibilities: the patient does not have the disease or infection or the pathogen is present but not in a high enough concentration for detection; this further explains discordant results between NAAT and antigen methods and the rationale for why negative antigen results should be reflexed for confirmation. Commercially available POC antigen tests should provide guidance on indications for confirmatory testing of possible false-negatives or, in some scenarios, suspected false-positive results. POC laboratories may have limited capacity to run such confirmatory assays, which are often referred out to larger commercial laboratories. Confirmatory testing also allows for evaluation of discordant results, changes to patient care plans, and insight into general test performance in your patient population.

Staff Training/Competency

Simple POC assays such as urine-based pregnancy tests, urinalysis by dipstick method, rapid SARS-CoV-2, rapid influenza, respiratory syncytial virus (RSV), GAS, and simple blood glucose tests are easy to use and familiar to many POC laboratory and clinical staff. Although the analytes and specimens may be different, the same principle of application of a clinical sample to a lateral flow chamber and waiting for development of a positive and control line are easily understood by most personnel at POC laboratories, such as urgent care clinics, physician office laboratories, or hospital wards. Despite some subjectivity on "positive" versus "negative" lines, these simplified kits decrease the perception of user-error concerns and minimize troubleshooting steps.

Costs

Antigen tests are historically much cheaper than molecular tests and require simplistic integration instruments, if one is required at all. Many antigen tests are less than $10 USD, and many purchasing contracts will include necessary equipment, such as an optical analyzer, without additional charge. In contrast, the cost of a single molecular run has decreased significantly, yet the cost per analyte still remains higher than an antigen test. The CMS 2022 Q4 Clinical Laboratory Fee Schedule reimbursement rates are between 2.1 and 6.8 times higher for NAAT than antigen methods (**Table 2**). These increased reimbursement rates are intended to defray additional costs associated with performance of molecular assays, including analyzer instrument

Table 1
Assay parameters of select commercially available point-of-care antigen diagnostic assays

Assay	Manufacturer	Specimen Source	Sensitivity (%)	Specificity (%)
QuickVue Dipstick Strep A Test	Quidel	Throat swab	92[a]	98[a]
QuickVue Influenza A + B Test	Quidel	Nasal/Nasopharyngeal (NP) swab	81.5/80.9[b]	97.8/99.1[b]
QuickVue SARS Antigen Test	Quidel	Nares swab	96.8[c]	99.1[c]
Determine HIV-1/2 Ag/Ab Combo Test	Abbott	Fingerstick whole blood	99.9[d]	99.8[d]
QuickVue RSV Test	Quidel	NP aspirate/NP/Nasal wash/NP wash	99/92/83[e]	92/92/90[e]
BinaxNOW *Streptococcus pneumoniae*				
Antigen Card	Abbott	Urine, CSF	86/97[f]	94/99[f]
BinaxNOW Legionella Urinary				
Antigen Card	Abbott	Urine	95[g]	95[g]
OSOM Trichomonas Rapid Test	SEKISUI Diagnostics	Vaginal swab	83[h]	99[h]
Immunocard Stat! Giardia	Meridian	Stool	100[i]	100[i]

[a] Compared with bacterial culture.
[b] Compared with molecular assay. Sensitivity and specificity for influenza A and influenza B, respectively.
[c] Compared with molecular EUA assay. Sensitivity and specificity for fresh specimens.
[d] Compared with patients who had tested positive/negative with enzyme immunoassay (EIA)/western blot.
[e] Compared with RSV culture. Sensitivity and specificity for nasopharyngeal (NP) aspirate/NP/nasal wash and NP wash, respectively, for pediatric patients.
[f] Compared with blood culture positive and negative patients and cerebrospinal fluid (CSF)-positive and -negative patients. Sensitivity and specificity for urine and CSF sources, respectively.
[g] Compared with archived positive and negative patient urine specimens.
[h] Compared with composite reference standard (wet mount and culture).
[i] Compared with microscopic reference standard. Product insert provides disclaimer that the relative comparison assay and no judgment can be made on the comparison assay's accuracy to predict disease.

Table 2					
Comparison of Centers for Medicare and Medicaid Services clinical laboratory fee schedule for antigen and molecular diagnostic assay[a]					
	Antigen		Molecular		
Assay	CPT Code[b]	Reimbursement Amount	CPT Code[c]	Reimbursement Amount	Fold Increase
RSV	87420	$13.91	87634	$70.20	5.1
Influenza A/B	87400	$14.13	87502	$95.80	6.8
Group A Strep	87430	$16.84	87651	$35.09	2.1
Trichomonas	87808	$15.29	87661	$35.09	2.3

[a] Based on publicly available 2022 quarter 4 laboratory fee schedule for clinical laboratories (www.cms.gov). This table is for illustrative purposes only and each laboratory must independently verify proper CPT code for their technology and assay employment.
[b] Current procedural terminology (CPT) codes are based on the waived (QW) designation using an instrument for detection and result interpretation.
[c] Molecular CPT code based on amplified probe technique.

maintenance, warranties, and ancillary consumables, along with potential cold storage requirements.

Time-to-Result and Time-to-Diagnosis

Time-to-result influences the decision to choose an antigen or a molecular-based assay. Most antigen detection assays result at 15 to 25 minutes where modern commercial NAAT assays typically require a minimum of 20 to 45 minutes to complete. Commercial manufacturers continue to optimize the timing of molecular assays for POC testing, and some molecular assays include early termination of testing cycles with results as soon as the molecular target is detected. Although this may equalize the time to positivity between methods for a positive result, a negative NAAT will not be reported until all amplification cycles have completed; this is to ensure there is no late amplification in cases of low copy numbers. Although this delay may be beneficial during high disease prevalence and decreases the requirement for reflex to confirmatory testing, delayed results may affect patient care flow in busy patient care settings.

Additional concerns of molecular platform implementation include the potential of backlog in patient testing because, to justify cost, only a single polymerase chain reaction (PCR) analyzer capable of performing testing on one to a few specimens at a time is likely. this limits how many specimens a laboratory can process at one time, increasing the time-to-result while decreasing the patient and provider satisfaction.

Laboratory Infrastructure

Molecular POC assays require meticulous handling and processing to reduce contamination and subsequent risk of inaccurate (primarily false-positive) results.

Potential sources of contamination include the reuse of disposable laboratory coats, failure to change gloves between samples, and opening more than one sample at a time. Environmental barriers such as biosafety cabinets to limit air currents are paramount to prevent cross-contamination. Personnel must be properly and routinely trained to ensure adherence with these procedures. Good laboratory practices dictate the same care should be present during antigen testing; however, the higher limit of detection and lack of amplified product will often mask low-level contamination not afforded to molecular methodology. Other infrastructure concerns include too few or poorly located electrical outlets, inadequate benchtop space, and lack of LIS/EHR integration.

Detecting Multiple Etiologic Agents

Another significant advantage of molecular-based assays is the ability to perform one test and return multiple results of 2 or more pathogenic agents. The presentation of the patient and medical history may help the provider elucidate the most likely pathogen but this is more difficult when symptoms and exposure to multiple circulating infectious agents is possible; this is especially true during respiratory viral season when influenza, SARS-CoV-2, respiratory syncytial virus, parainfluenza, adenovirus, and rhinovirus/enterovirus can all present with similar symptoms. Although treatment may not be altered by testing outcome, the impact on public health, isolation of the patient, and insight into secondary complications is medically necessary to the health care and local community alike.

The POC assays selected for these cases becomes important and leaves the provider with difficult decisions for additional testing if negative assay results only correlate to a single pathogen. Guidance from current epidemiology of circulating infectious agents and patient history may help but, when the differential diagnosis includes multiple pathogens, a POC multianalyte panel may be the best choice and no other testing methodology is robust as multitargeted PCR panels. Current POC PCR panels include a 19-target respiratory pathogen panel that detects common viral and bacterial agents and combinatory influenza and RSV panels.

SPECIFIC ASSAY CONSIDERATIONS
Group A Streptococcus

GAS (Streptococcus pyogenes) is a common pathogen, and POC testing for this organism is frequently an antigen-based throat swab. A meta-analysis from 2014 identified GAS antigen testing had a pooled sensitivity of 86% (95% confidence interval [CI] of 83%–88%) and specificity of 96% (95 CI of 94%–97%). Increased sensitivity is gained by molecular methods without a change in collection methods or specimen source. A major benefit of NAAT detection of GAS is that secondary culture-based testing to confirm false-negative antigen testing is not required.[11] Because of the analytical target for S pyogenes remains relatively stable compared with other etiologic agents, such as viral targets, the choice of antigen versus molecular is condensed to best patient care and reimbursement rate.

Influenza

Influenza virus types A and B are considered cyclic, seasonal infections. Although antigen assays and most molecular waived POC option detect presence and absence of each influenza virus type A and B, Biofire Diagnostics (Salt Lake City, UT, USA) currently offers a waived multianalyte NAAT that will report subtypes. If a POC laboratory is licensed to perform assays registered by the Food and Drug Administration as moderate-complexity, additional commercial assays that will report subtype are available. Viral subtype detection is important to assist providers and public health professionals in determination of infection risk and early detection of novel strains that may have crossed zoonotic lines. Each year, as people are vaccinated against the predicted dominant strains of influenza, a knowledge of the circulating subtypes in the local community and the impact to the assay's performance is beneficial.

Viral detection by molecular and antigen method performance can be influenced by the viral subtype and, if a variant arises, may limit the ability of the assays, with the antigen assay being most negatively affected. This case was demonstrated in 2009 with the novel influenza H1N1 outbreak. The accuracy of the antigen assay was reduced to 37.8% due to a high false-positive rate, sensitivity was estimated as low as 17.8% compared with the molecular assay with a sensitivity of 97.8%, and the specificity was estimated between 48.1% and 50.7%. [12–15]

SARS-CoV-2

Molecular testing for SARS-CoV-2 is best for both patient care and public health prevention; however, the inability of some clinics to implement molecular testing or inability of a patient to be seen by a health care provider lends initial screening to antigen testing as a matter of convenience. Although POC and home-test COVID antigen assays are abundant, the assay's performance in terms of sensitivity and high limit-of-detection favors the molecular test method for early detection. Antigen testing for SARS-CoV-2 peaks 4 to 5 days after symptom onset, and a direct comparison of antigen to NAAT favored molecular methods for earlier detection of SARS-CoV-2 compared with antigenic methods if both are performed in tandem. [6,16]

Although molecular assays have higher sensitivity and can identify early infection and drive initial isolation decisions and public health response, the overall selection of antigen or molecular tests is dependent on the medical indication and progress of disease. The COVID19 pandemic illustrated this concept well, as early detection was best done using molecular methods but could not determine the risk of shedding long-term infectious virus due to assay detection of remnant, noninfectious viral RNA. [17] The antigen test, however, has a delay in positivity rate. Reports are varied on conducting antigen testing after a positive result as a predictor of active of infectious viral shedding. A few studies suggest a positive antigen result during or after symptom resolution is a marker of infectious viral shedding but evidence is limited and current guidance by the Infectious Disease Society of America has not endorsed this viewpoint because there is too few clinical trials and studies to make a strong claim. [18–21] Together, guidance from public health officials has evolved from early testing algorithms to suggest molecular testing should not be used to guide long-term isolation decisions and symptom resolution after isolation is sufficient for predicting contagiousness. Current Centers for Disease Control and Prevention (CDC) guidance only suggests an individual who has resolved symptoms can discontinue masking before 10 days if their symptoms are resolved and 2 antigen tests, conducted at least 48 hours apart, are negative. [22] Overall, the best strategy for early COVID19 detection is using a molecular-based method for recent onset of symptoms, but, to confirm resolution, a negative result based on antigen methods or waiting the minimum of 10 days after symptom onset is recommended.

Human Immunodeficiency Virus

Fourth-generation human immunodeficiency virus (HIV) testing that incorporates detection of the p24 antigen is one of the most common antigen tests on the market. Sensitivity of an HIV antigen test is sufficiently high at time of a symptomatic patient presentation that current practices only use molecular methods for confirmation and treatment response. Rarely is a false-negative a concern of HIV p24 rapid antigen POC tests with symptomatic patients due to the assay's high sensitivity; however, the assay has many false-positives due to its lowered specificity, and, like other sexually acquired infections, the time-to-diagnosis is essential in reducing public health impact through community spread. Because false-positives are far more common with the p24 antigen test, confirmatory testing by NAAT is a necessity. Currently, no point-of-care molecular test for HIV is available but the risk of false-negatives and effects is significant that false-positive antigen testing followed by confirmation using molecular is best suited for the POC setting.

Respiratory Syncytial Virus

In the recent decade, molecular testing for RSV has increased in outpatient setting but remain stable in emergency departments and in-patient settings.[23] Although data presented from national databases on RSV positivity seem that antigen testing is more accurate than PCR, this is not the case because most PCR tests are done as a confirmatory test of a negative antigen and most RSV positive patients have been screened out before PCR testing. The national database data also suggest the reason why molecular testing has not increased in the in-patient and emergency departments is that those healthcare POC settings are less likely to reflex a negative test than outpatient settings.

Sensitivity comparisons between antigen and molecular methods clearly support molecular methods for all demographics but especially in adult populations. A meta-analysis found sensitivity of antigen testing in pediatric populations was 81% (95% CI, 78%–84%) compared with adults at 29% (95% CI 11%–48%).[24] Another study published in 2022 found that specimens collected on the same patient during presentation to an emergency room found that use of PCR methods more than doubled diagnosis of RSV.[25] Considering the assay performance, molecular testing is still best for patient diagnosis but the associated costs and management of patients in these 3 distinct health care environments may sway testing protocols.

Current POC RSV molecular assays are combined with other respiratory illnesses, most notably influenza. In children younger than 6 years, RSV was detected with influenza or human metapneumovirus more often than other age groups, suggesting the risk of coinfection was greatest in pediatric patients.[26] For this age group, a strong consideration for multianalyte molecular testing is warranted compared with a nonpediatric demographic where the single-analyte antigen assays carry less likelihood of excluding an additional diagnosis due to coinfection.

Streptococcus pneumoniae

Streptococcus pneumoniae is a common pathogen responsible for community-acquired pneumonia. A 27-study meta-analysis of the S pneumoniae urine antigen assay found a sensitivity of 74% and specificity of 97.2% relative to culture methods.[27] Current antigen assays on the market result at 15 minutes compared with NAATs, which are greater than 1 hour. Initial, single gene targeted NAAT assays were lackluster with detection rates as low as 62%.[28] As other gene targets were challenged, sensitivities improved but the question of positive prediction value was questioned, as S pneumoniae can be a commensal organism at low concentrations but pathogenic at elevated amounts. Currently, there is only one commercial, moderate-complexity NAAT option on market that distinguishes between the intensity of gene amplification product to determine commensal versus pathogenic states.[29]

This multianalyte molecular panel uses sputum or bronchoalveolar lavage, leaving many POC settings to choose the antigen test by necessity of cost, easier specimen collection, and processing advantages. Although the convenience of antigen testing for POC environment outweighs NAAT options, false-negatives compared with positive blood or sputum cultures are still prevalent.[30] Other Streptococcus species also cross-react with the urine antigen test causing false-positives, especially if used to diagnosis S pneumoniae in children.[31] Together, although the urine antigen test may be an attractive option, the limitations of result accuracy warrants consideration of removal of the POC test in favor for molecular methods, even at the cost of time for reference laboratory testing.

Legionella pneumophila

Legionellosis can be diagnosed by NAAT using sputum as the source; however, urine antigen testing is the only available option in a Clinical Laboratory Improvement Amendments of 1988 (CLIA)-waived registered POC setting where both multipanel analyte NAAT methods and urine antigen methods can be used in a POC setting registered to perform moderate-complexity assays.[32] Antigen testing provides easier specimen collection and lower cost in a POC setting compared with NAAT; however, considering the rarity of Legionella and patient presentation between Legionellosis and other bacterial causes of pneumonia, a provider suspecting Legionella should strongly consider a multianalyte molecular panel over the antigen test. One multicenter study found a false-negative rate of greater than 44% of the urine antigen test, leading to a missed diagnosis in 39% of the patient population.[33] Fortunately, few providers develop a differential diagnosis that includes Legionellosis as a primary concern, and, therefore, few POC locations stock the urine antigen tests and prefer to send out to reference for multianalyte testing.

Trichomonas vaginalis

Trichomonas vaginalis is a parasite implicated in the sexually transmitted infection trichomoniasis. Commercial POC antigen assays are widely available, and some providers choose to diagnosis T vaginalis by wet mount microscopy despite the low sensitivity.[34] To fill this gap, Trichomonas antigen testing was introduced in the mid-1980s and became the preference of many waived POC laboratories with increased sensitivities compared with microscopy of greater than 90%; however, this increase is misleading considering the insensitivity of microscopy.[35] When the antigen assay is compared with a composite comparator of microscopic method and culture, the sensitivity increases to 83% to 86% largely due to culture methods, which are not routinely performed in reference clinical settings. Molecular assays compared with antigen methods demonstrate sensitivities between 98% and 100% but these are only available to laboratories registered to perform nonwaived testing.[36] Recently, in addition to the commonly tested genital or rectal specimens, requests to diagnosis T vaginalis from pharyngeal specimens are increasing, largely due to the low limits of detection and high sensitivity of the molecular assays. Although inclusion of pharyngeal specimens for molecular sexually transmitted infection (STI) testing opens capabilities for increased diagnostic capabilities over antigen testing, this area must be studied more, as cross-reactivity with other organisms present in the upper respiratory tract may lead to false-positives.[37] Although the barrier to implement a molecular testing platform may seem daunting for a small POC clinic and require nonwaived testing registration, the impact on STI diagnosis would benefit patients, providers, and public health.

Giardia

Giardia detection was traditionally performed by microscopic means but was labor- and time-intensive with potential low sensitivity due to the expertise required for parasitic identification. Specificity was high for the genus but speciation for public health needs was not possible. Antigen testing improved sensitivity for the general testing personnel compared with microscopic methods and greatly reduced time-to-result, helping to diminish outbreak potential. Although specificity remained suboptimal, some early reports show sensitivity as high as 94% compared with microscopic methods but other studies suggest much lower sensitivity such as 60.7% during a waterborne outbreak case.[38,39] Although antigen detection enabled POC settings to perform testing, the CDC still recommends testing 3 stool samples over the course of several days to increase antigen result accuracy. Because most POC settings do not lend to multiple patient visits, the utility of the *Giardia* antigen test and proper use is questionable when molecular options demonstrate improved sensitivity and specificity and one sample is considered diagnostic.

PERSONAL PERSPECTIVES AND FUTURE PROSPECTS

Antigen testing revolutionized the ability to diagnosis, accurately prescribe, and track local epidemiology within the POC setting. Antigen testing is relatively low cost, does not require sophisticated instrumentation, is portable, and can easily be implemented in both first- and third-world POC scenarios. As convenient as antigen testing is, there are drawbacks in the time-to-initial-diagnosis postsymptom onset due to lower limit of detection, sensitivity, and, occasionally, specificity that molecular options overcome. Alas, only a few POC-waived molecular options are currently in the US market, with some laboratories opting to elevate their CLIA registration to moderate complexity to perform molecular tests in the POC setting. As NAAT testing becomes more familiar to health care clinics and the public, and impeding operational costs and implementation are overcome, there will be an increased demand for these molecular assays and a shift away from their antigen counterpart in POC settings. Although molecular testing offers a greater prospect for definitive diagnosis and patient care, they will not fully replace antigen tests in the POC setting in the near future unless overhead and testing costs are reduced and more commercial options for waived molecular options are developed.

A longer-term future prospect of antigen assays is a shift from the POC setting to at-home testing. The release of at-home COVID-19 antigen assays during the pandemic raises the question if antigen assays could be primarily used in the home testing environment while molecular assays remain exclusive to the health care setting. The implications are still early and highly debatable. At-home antigen testing and interpterion would require significant public education by public health experts and providers. Nonetheless, antigen tests will always have a role in the health care system but only the future will determine the degree that molecular tests will dominant the POC setting and drive an at-home testing if antigen tests become more available.

CLINICS CARE POINTS

- Antigen-based diagnostic assays are often similar in specificity to molecular assays but have a lower sensitivity which increases the risk of false-negative results.
- Negative antigen test results should be confirmed by a molecular assay, especially if the patient is presenting early with symptoms, the prevalence of the infectious agent is high, or the infection is high on the differential diagnosis.
- Positive HIV antigen test results, should always be confirmed by a secondary testing method, commonly a molecular assay, due to potential false-positives and to delineate between types of HIV strains that can impact treatment decisions.
- Antigen and molecular assay vary between the time-to-detection and how long the infectious agent can be detected. Ensure to select the correct assay type based on symptom onset and the objective of testing.
- Some molecular assays may remain positive after the patient symptoms have resolved. Consultation with an infectious disease provider, board-certified medical microbiologist, or epidemiologist may help determine clinical significance.

DISCLOSURES

The authors declare no relevant or material financial interests related to this publication.

REFERENCES

1. Mabey D, Peeling RW, Ustianowski A, et al. Diagnostics for the developing world. Nat Rev Microbiol 2004;2:231–40.
2. Naseri M, Ziora ZM, Simon GP, et al. ASSURED-compliant point-of-care diagnostics for the detection of human viral infections. Rev Med Virol 2022;32:2263.
3. Kettler H, White K, Hawkes S. 2004. Mapping the landscape of diagnostics for sexually transmitted infections: Key findings and recommandations. UNICEF/UNDP/World Bank/WHO. World Health Organization.
4. Otoo JA, Schlappi TS. REASSURED multiplex diagnostics: a critical review and forecast. Biosensors (Basel) 2022;12.
5. Peeling RW, Mabey D. Point-of-care tests for diagnosing infections in the developing world. Clin Microbiol Infect 2010;16:1062–9.
6. Chu VT, Schwartz NG, Donnelly MAP, et al. Comparison of home antigen testing with RT-PCR and viral culture during the course of SARS-CoV-2 infection. JAMA Intern Med 2022;182:701–9.
7. Azar MM, Landry ML. Detection of influenza A and B viruses and respiratory syncytial virus by use of clinical laboratory improvement amendments of 1988 (CLIA)-Waived point-of-care assays: a paradigm shift to molecular tests. J Clin Microbiol 2018;56.
8. Drexler JF, Helmer A, Kirberg H, et al. Poor clinical sensitivity of rapid antigen test for influenza A pandemic (H1N1) 2009 virus. Emerg Infect Dis 2009;15:1662–4.
9. Uhl JR, Adamson SC, Vetter EA, et al. Comparison of LightCycler PCR, rapid antigen immunoassay, and culture for detection of group A streptococci from throat swabs. J Clin Microbiol 2003;41:242–9.
10. Arnaout R, Lee RA, Lee GR, et al. The limit of detection matters: the case for benchmarking severe acute respiratory syndrome coronavirus 2 testing. Clin Infect Dis 2021;73:e3042–6.
11. Lean WL, Arnup S, Danchin M, et al. Rapid diagnostic tests for group A streptococcal pharyngitis: a meta-analysis. Pediatrics 2014;134:771–81.
12. Ginocchio CC, Zhang F, Manji R, et al. Evaluation of multiple test methods for the detection of the novel 2009 influenza A (H1N1) during the New York City outbreak. J Clin Virol 2009;45:191–5.
13. Stevenson HL, Loeffelholz MJ. Poor positive accuracy of QuickVue rapid antigen tests during the influenza A (H1N1) 2009 pandemic. J Clin Microbiol 2010;48:3729–31.
14. Sambol AR, Abdalhamid B, Lyden ER, et al. Use of rapid influenza diagnostic tests under field conditions as a screening tool during an outbreak of the 2009 novel influenza virus: practical considerations. J Clin Virol 2010;47:229–33.
15. Likitnukul S, Boonsiri K, Tangsuksant Y. Evaluation of sensitivity and specificity of rapid influenza diagnostic tests for novel swine-origin influenza A (H1N1) virus. Pediatr Infect Dis J 2009;28:1038–9.
16. Mina MJ, Parker R, Larremore DB. Rethinking covid-19 test sensitivity - a strategy for containment. N Engl J Med 2020;383:e120.
17. Binnicker MJ. Can testing predict SARS-CoV-2 infectivity? The potential for certain methods to Be surrogates for replication-competent virus. J Clin Microbiol 2021;59. 004699-e521.

18. Lopera TJ, Alzate-Ángel JC, Díaz FJ, et al. The usefulness of antigen testing in predicting contagiousness in COVID-19. Microbiol Spectr 2022;10. 019622-e2021.
19. Hayden M.K., Hanson K.E., Englund J.A., et al., 2022. Infectious diseases society of America guidelines on the diagnosis of COVID-19: antigen testing., on infectious diseases society of America. Available at: https://www.idsociety.org/practice-guideline/covid-19-guideline-antigen-testing/. Accessed January 16th, 2023.
20. Puhach O, Meyer B, Eckerle I. SARS-CoV-2 viral load and shedding kinetics. Nat Rev Microbiol 2022. https://doi.org/10.1038/s41579-022-00822-w.
21. Fotouhi F, Salehi-Vaziri M, Farahmand B, et al. Prolonged viral shedding and antibody persistence in patients with COVID-19. Microbes Infect 2021;23:104810.
22. Centers for Disease Control and Prevention. 2022. Guidance for antigen testing for SARS-CoV-2 for healthcare providers testing individuals in the community. Available at: https://www.cdc.gov/coronavirus/2019-ncov/lab/resources/antigen-tests-guidelines.html. Accessed January 16th, 2023.
23. Tran PT, Nduaguba SO, Diaby V, et al. RSV testing practice and positivity by patient demographics in the United States: integrated analyses of MarketScan and NREVSS databases. BMC Infect Dis 2022;22:681.
24. Chartrand C, Tremblay N, Renaud C, et al. Diagnostic accuracy of rapid antigen detection tests for respiratory syncytial virus infection: systematic review and meta-analysis. J Clin Microbiol 2015;53:3738–49.
25. Yin N, Van Nuffelen M, Bartiaux M, et al. Clinical impact of the rapid molecular detection of RSV and influenza A and B viruses in the emergency department. PLOS ONE 2022;17:e0274222.
26. Ramaekers K, Keyaerts E, Rector A, et al. Prevalence and seasonality of six respiratory viruses during five consecutive epidemic seasons in Belgium. J Clin Virol 2017;94:72–8.
27. Sinclair A, Xie X, Teltscher M, et al. Systematic review and meta-analysis of a urine-based pneumococcal antigen test for diagnosis of community-acquired pneumonia caused by Streptococcus pneumoniae. J Clin Microbiol 2013;51:2303–10.
28. Peters RP, de Boer RF, Schuurman T, et al. Streptococcus pneumoniae DNA load in blood as a marker of infection in patients with community-acquired pneumonia. J Clin Microbiol 2009;47:3308–12.
29. Webber DM, Wallace MA, Burnham CA, et al. Evaluation of the BioFire FilmArray pneumonia panel for detection of viral and bacterial pathogens in lower respiratory tract specimens in the setting of a tertiary care academic medical center. J Clin Microbiol 2020;58.
30. Smith MD, Sheppard CL, Hogan A, et al. Diagnosis of Streptococcus pneumoniae infections in adults with bacteremia and community-acquired pneumonia: clinical comparison of pneumococcal PCR and urinary antigen detection. J Clin Microbiol 2009;47:1046–9.
31. Ghaffar F, Friedland IR, McCracken GH Jr. Dynamics of nasopharyngeal colonization by Streptococcus pneumoniae. Pediatr Infect Dis J 1999;18:638–46.
32. Bencini MA, van den Brule AJ, Claas EC, et al. Multicenter comparison of molecular methods for detection of Legionella spp. in sputum samples. J Clin Microbiol 2007;45:3390–2.
33. Muyldermans A, Descheemaeker P, Boel A, et al, On behalf of the National Expert Committee on Infectious S. What is the risk of missing legionellosis relying on urinary antigen testing solely? A retrospective Belgian multicenter study. Eur J Clin Microbiol Infect Dis 2020;39:729–34.

34. Bruni MP, Freitas da Silveira M, Stauffert D, et al. Aptima Trichomonas vaginalis assay elucidates significant underdiagnosis of trichomoniasis among women in Brazil according to an observational study. Sex Transm Infect 2019;95:129–32.
35. Sekisui D. 2013. OSOM Trichomonas Rapid Test, vol Rev. 3084-1, San Diego, CA.
36. Gaydos CA, Klausner JD, Pai NP, et al. Rapid and point-of-care tests for the diagnosis of Trichomonas vaginalis in women and men. Sex Transm Infect 2017;93:S31–5.
37. Chesnay A, Pastuszka A, Richard L, et al. Multiplex PCR assay targeting Trichomonas vaginalis: need for biological evaluation and interpretation. Diagn Microbiol Infect Dis 2022;104:115808.
38. Strand EA, Robertson LJ, Hanevik K, et al. Sensitivity of a Giardia antigen test in persistent giardiasis following an extensive outbreak. Clin Microbiol Infect 2008; 14:1069–71.
39. Garcia LS, Shimizu RY, Novak S, et al. Commercial assay for detection of *Giardia lamblia* and *Cryptosporidium parvum* antigens in human fecal specimens by rapid solid-phase qualitative immunochromatography. J Clin Microbiol 2003;41: 209–12.

The Role of Point-of-Care Testing in Specific Populations

Nicholas Yared, MD

KEYWORDS

- Point-of-care tests • Rapid diagnostic tests • HIV • Rural health care • Mobile health

KEY POINTS

- Point-of-care testing (POCT) as defined by the ability to provide diagnostic sites at the site of patient care with rapid turnaround time is particularly beneficial for certain patient populations.
- Infectious conditions, such as HIV and hepatitis C, are particularly amenable to the use of point-of-care tests because rapid diagnostics can positively impact the cascade of care for these conditions.
- An understanding of a country's "diagnostic ecosystem," or how its health care systems is structured, its regulatory environment around testing, and how patients engage with the country's health care infrastructure, is essential for effective deployment of POCT for resource-limited settings.
- POCT provided at home or in mobile units is a frequently effective and acceptable method for using diagnostic tests in difficult-to-reach populations.
- Economic factors, laboratory and personnel infrastructure challenges, and health system–related factors allow for persistent gaps in POCT access and utilization in low- and middle-income countries compared with higher-income countries and between rural and urban regions. Multiple strategies, including leveraging of communication technologies, the use of mobile clinics, implementation of novel geospatial science concepts, and changes in national health care policy, can help reduce these gaps.

INTRODUCTION

The goal of point-of-care testing (POCT) is to provide medical testing at or near the site of patient care in order to improve outcomes by reducing turnaround time.[1] POCT has multiple advantages through decreasing caregiver inconvenience, diagnostic delays, and transportation costs.[2] It can also facilitate timely linkage to appropriate medical care and referral. Moreover, POCT has a role for providing testing during

Division of Infectious Diseases, Department of Medicine, Henry Ford Health, 2799 West Grand Boulevard, Detroit, MI 48202, USA
E-mail address: nyared1@hfhs.org

Clin Lab Med 43 (2023) 181–187
https://doi.org/10.1016/j.cll.2023.02.004
0272-2712/23/© 2023 Elsevier Inc. All rights reserved.
labmed.theclinics.com

events, such as natural disasters or pandemics, when patients may be constrained from accessing traditional clinic settings. A survey conducted by the University of Massachusetts of 277 participants regarding POCT during the COVID-19 pandemic found that 94% of respondents agreed or strongly agreed that POCT could improve their care. In addition, the majority of respondents reported having POCT in their home setting as a top priority.[3]

Whether POCT is used varies among different medical settings and patient populations. Historically, the development of POCT was driven by the need for testing or monitoring of the health status of particular populations often outside of traditional health care settings where quick results were needed. For example, home blood glucose monitors were developed in the 1970s to assist patients with insulin dose adjustments.[4] Urgent care settings often do not have an on-site laboratory, and POCT can assist with the assessment and management of commonly encountered conditions. In traditional ambulatory care clinics, POCT has the ability to provide rapid testing to screen for common conditions, test for simple syndromes with limited differential diagnoses, and provide frequent monitoring for certain therapies (eg, anticoagulation).[5]

Understanding the context in which POCT is deployed is necessary to determine which specific populations may receive the greatest benefit from its use. This article illustrates particular populations in whom the use of point-of-care tests evolved and for whom POCT can mitigate or overcome barriers specific to these groups when seeking medical care.

POINT-OF-CARE TESTING FOR SPECIFIC POPULATIONS: THE EXAMPLE OF PEOPLE LIVING WITH HUMAN IMMUNODEFICIENCY VIRUS

One patient population in particular that serves to illustrate the advantages and limitations of POCT is people living with HIV (PLWH). Although the incidence of HIV has been gradually decreasing in the United States, 34,800 incident cases of HIV occurred in 2019.[6] PLWH who have achieved viral suppression (<200 copies HIV RNA per milliliter) have no risk of transmitting the virus; however, 38% of new HIV infections occur from individuals unaware of their diagnosis who had not undergone testing, and 43% of new HIV infections occur from individuals previously diagnosed with HIV but out of medical care.[7]

Given the necessity to identify individuals living with HIV and monitor their viral suppression once diagnosed, methods to promote testing for HIV are key to control the epidemic. The US Department of Health and Human Services developed the Ending the HIV Epidemic plan with a goal to work with local communities to diagnose, treat, and prevent HIV as well as to respond to potential HIV outbreaks. Overall, the goal of the program is to reduce the number of new HIV infections by at least 75% by 2025 and by at least 90% by 2030 with increased testing being a crucial component to achieving these goals.[8] The Centers for Disease Control and Prevention (CDC) has also recommended since 2006 that persons disproportionately impacted by HIV, such as men who have sex with men (MSM), get tested for HIV annually.[9,10]

HIV self-testing using a rapid point-of-care test, the OraQuick in-home HIV test (OraSure Technologies, Inc., Bethlehem, PA, USA), has been investigated as an option for increasing the outreach of HIV testing.[11,12] The OraQuick test was approved as an over-the-counter home-based HIV test by the US Food and Drug Administration in July 2012.[13] A prior review of HIV self-testing highlighted common barriers associated with the use of home point-of-care tests, including financial issues owing to the cost of testing and limited availability of research data to support the benefit of self-administered POCT for HIV.[14] However, a randomized controlled trial evaluating the use of HIV self-testing using oral fluid HIV self-tests compared with usual testing performed at community sites among high-risk MSM in Seattle, Washington demonstrated significantly increased tests performed over a 15-month period among the self-testing group using POCT (mean, 5.3; CI, 4.7–6) compared with those who underwent testing as usual (mean, 3.6; CI, 1.9–2.7).[12]

Similarly, during the COVID-19 pandemic, the CDC deployed the use of TakeMeHome, a centralized system for distributing HIV self-test kits using oral fluid POCT. Over the course of 12 months, 5325 kits were mailed to 4904 persons with 36% of recipients reporting never having tested for HIV. Among 855 respondents to a follow-up survey, 90% were willing to recommend the program to a friend, 63% thought that the program addressed issues of convenience, and 46% thought that it addressed issues of privacy. In addition, greater than 10% of participants sought other HIV and sexually transmitted infection prevention services following use of the HIV self-test.[11] These findings highlight the potential for home POCT to reach individuals who may not present to traditional clinic settings. They also demonstrate high levels of acceptability of self-testing using point-of-care tests. However, both studies focused primarily on MSM, potentially limiting their generalizability to other populations. Moreover, documentation of test results and linkage to care and follow-up in clinic settings were not tracked, and these remain ongoing challenges with self-administered point-of-care tests.

USAGE OF POINT-OF-CARE TESTING IN RURAL AND RESOURCE-LIMITED SETTINGS

Populations living in rural regions and resource-limited settings may particularly benefit from the use of POCT given that timely results can facilitate linkage to care and quick initiation of appropriate therapies. However, several barriers to the adoption of POCT exists in these settings. Practicing clinicians working in resource-limited settings may prefer a syndromic approach to clinical presentations rather than the single disease focus involved with many point-of-care tests. Moreover, clinicians may also prioritize the use of empiric therapy for managing syndromic conditions rather than using POCT to achieve diagnostic certainty. In addition, quality assurance of testing and operator experience can be limited in these settings. The rural workforce is often not laboratory-trained and may be unfamiliar with or lack the capacity to perform quality assurance on available point-of-care tests. Finally, the decision to use certain POCT may be influenced by concerns around trust of the health care system and stigma with certain results (eg, HIV testing) based on the receptive population's cultural practices and preferences.

An understanding of a population's engagement with their health care system and the regulatory frameworks around POCT is crucial to using it in a way that leverages its benefits and overcomes testing barriers. One example of this "diagnostic ecosystem" is the use of rapid diagnostic tests (RDTs) for testing for infectious conditions in India. There are a variety of infectious RDTs available for use in India with these tests being relatively inexpensive. However, a review of the state of POCT there revealed that most testing still took place in hospitals and laboratories with little utilization in homes, community-based venues, or clinics. In addition, incentives in place for private doctors to use POCT with uneven quality assurance testing has resulted in the proliferation of some inaccurate diagnostics, including tuberculosis serology before the banning of its use by the government.[15]

Lack of governmental regulation of POCT is also a problem that can disproportionately impact populations living in rural or remote areas because of concerns about the quality of testing. However, governments are increasingly taking steps to put forward regulatory legislation to address this issue. One significant example is the Therapeutic Products Bill in New Zealand. This legislation has been put forward to provide a comprehensive regulatory framework for point-of-care medical testing devices that would greatly improve product safety standards, particularly in rural and remote regions of New Zealand.[16]

Communication and information technologies can be leveraged to overcoming some of the challenges with using POCT in remote and resource-limited settings. Mobile phone technology has allowed for automatic data capture from POCT, remote reporting and counseling about results, and a method for external quality assurance. It can also serve as a decision support system for clinicians to assist with interpretation of POCT results.[15] Mobile health units to provide POCT have also demonstrated promise in overcoming infrastructure challenges for difficult-to-reach populations and those in rural and resource-limited settings. An illustrative example is a study that used rapid hepatitis C antibody and RNA tests in Spain to impact the hepatitis C virus (HCV) cascade of care among groups at elevated risk, including persons who inject drugs (PWID), unhoused populations, and persons with mental health or alcohol use disorders. Among 214 individuals diagnosed with HCV at the mobile unit, 83.1% followed up at a hospital for evaluation for treatment, 76.6% started HCV treatment, and 65.8% completed therapy with almost all individuals completing therapy (95.2%), achieving sustained virologic response and HCV cure.[17] Although certain groups of individuals (eg, PWID) were less likely to progress along the care cascade to HCV cure, this study serves as an example of integrating POCT into an emerging model of care to bring testing to difficult-to-reach populations.

ENDURING GAPS IN POINT-OF-CARE TEST ACCESS

Although the use of POCT for certain infectious conditions has increased over time, gaps in the availability of other POCT targets remains an issue in particular areas. A recent systematic scoping review evaluating the use of patient self-testing in low- and middle-income countries (LMICs) demonstrated a lack of self-testing assays for noncommunicable diseases in these countries with 7 out of 8 of the articles analyzed dealing with HIV testing.[18] In contrast, analysis of the use of POCT assays for noncommunicable conditions, such as diabetes mellitus or anticoagulation monitoring, has been more robust in high-income countries.[19,20]

Several factors likely account for the discrepancy in the availability of POCT for noncommunicable diseases and neglected tropical diseases in LMICs. Development of point-of-care tests typically occurs in highly resourced countries with robust research infrastructure, which leads to a disconnect between where devices are developed and manufactured and where they are most needed. In addition, POCT developers focused on their return of investment from their products may be disincentivized to develop tests for neglected tropical diseases or to distribute tests used for common noncommunicable conditions to more rural and remote regions.[21] Pricing of point-of-care tests may also be unaffordable for many individuals residing in LMICs, limiting their availability and utilization.[15]

In addition to economic limitations, concerns related to available infrastructure, personnel, and training can also impact POCT utilization. The "ASSURED" criteria were originally developed by the World Health Organization as 7 core criteria that encapsulated characteristics of ideal diagnostic testing involving point-of-care assays (Affordable, Sensitive, Specific, User-friendly, Rapid and robust, Equipment-free or minimized, Deliverable).[22] However, application of these criteria in resource-limited settings can be particularly challenging given that a certain level of equipment and quality assurance training is still needed and may be lacking. Purchasing extra POCT materials for quality control and assurance poses a potential barrier for continued maintenance of high-quality POCT. In areas where materials are adequate, high staff turnover may still pose a challenge because of the lack of expertise in implementation and interpretation of tests.[21] Where adequately trained personnel and materials are available, point-of-care tests that are successfully obtained may face a final hurdle in their utility if there is a lack of additional laboratory infrastructure for monitoring and tracking of tests or a lack of individuals to provide posttest counseling for follow-up of their results.[15,21]

Addressing the gaps in the availability and use of POCT between urban areas in higher-income countries and rural and remote regions in lower-income countries will likely require reframing the goal of POCT. Although the ASSURED criteria outline an ideal framework for POCT that focuses on ease of testing and communication of results, some researchers have argued that a focus on the ability of POCT to facilitate linkage to long-term care is more useful for lower-resource settings.[23] Other methods to narrow the gap in POCT availability have focused on novel interventions for implementation, which often include solutions that have emerged in the context of disasters or crises. Mapping out small world networks, or well-connected topographically similar nodes and clusters of communities, can be a first step in strategically planning how to best distribute POCT infrastructure.[24] Utilization of geographic information systems, which are systems designed to create, store, and manage geographic data, can also be combined with POCT to optimize POCT use as illustrated by its application to the 2014 to 2015 Ebola outbreak in West Africa.[24,25] Finally, health care policy legislation at the national level, as previously noted with the example in New Zealand, can help lessen the inequities associated with POCT deployment in rural, remote, and lower-income settings.[16]

SUMMARY

Much of the emergence of POCT has been connected to the need to address barriers to care that are faced by specific patient populations. As previously noted, for certain groups, such as PLWH or PWID, the availability of point-of-care tests has allowed the flexibility to reach out to groups in venues outside of traditional medical facilities where patients are less likely to perceive care-related stigma.[11,12,17] For patient populations that have been difficult to reach because of their remoteness from traditional health care settings, POCT provides an option for diagnostic capability whereby home-based testing or pop-up or mobile clinics are used.[11,15,17]

Despite these advantages for specific patient populations, a continued understanding of the larger health care context in which point-of-care tests are deployed is needed to maximize their reach and benefit. Gaps in the availability of POCT in rural and remote settings and LMICs compared with more urban and higher-income countries result from a complex mix of economic factors, laboratory capacity and infrastructure issues, personnel issues, and health system–related factors.[15,21] Reframing the goal of POCT toward achievement of long-term linkage to care for underserved groups, support for POCT goals from national legislation, and the application of novel geospatial science methods to POCT implementation can help lessen POCT gaps.

DISCLOSURE

The author has nothing to disclose.

CLINICS CARE POINTS

- Deployment of rapid point-of-care self-tests for HIV and Hepatitis C detection can increase testing outreach and improve the HIV and Hepatitis C cascades of care.

- Mobile phone technology and mobile health units can be utilized to increase the availability of POCT in remote regions and improve access to POCT for difficult-to-reach populations.

- Clinicians can work with data scientists to understand how to best overcome barriers to access to POCT through the use of network mapping and utilization of geographic information systems.

- Clinician involvement with crafting national healthcare policy can decrease inequities in access to POCT for individuals living in rural, remote, and lower-income settings.

REFERENCES

1. Kost G. In: *Principles and practice of point-of-care testing.* Philadelphia, PA: Lippincott Williams & Wilkins; 2002. p. 654.
2. Parvin CA, Lo SF, Deuser SM, et al. Impact of point-of-care testing on patients' length of stay in a large emergency department. Clin Chem 1996;42(5):711–7.
3. Lilly CM, Ensom E, Teebagy S, et al. Patient preferences for point-of-care testing: survey validation and results. Point Care 2020;19(4):112–5.
4. Geffner ME, Kaplan SA, Lippe BM, et al. Self-monitoring of blood glucose levels and intensified insulin therapy: acceptability and efficacy in childhood diabetes. JAMA 1983;249:2913–6.
5. Peaper DR, Durant T, Campbell S. Distributed microbiology testing: Bringing infectious disease diagnostics to point of care. Clin Lab Med 2019;39:419–31.
6. Centers for Disease Control and Prevention. HIV surveillance report: estimated HIV incidence and prevalence in the United States, 2015-2019. Available at: https://www.cdc.gov/hiv/pdf/library/reports/surveillance/cdc-hiv-surveillance-supplemental-report-vol-26-1.pdf. Accessed October 30, 2022.
7. Li Z, Purcell DW, Sansom SL, et al. Vital signs: HIV transmission along the continuum of care—United States, 2016. MMWR Morb Mortal Wkly Rep 2019;68: 267–72. https://doi.org/10.15585/mmwr.mm6811e1.
8. Centers for Disease Control. Ending the HIV epidemic: a plan for America. Available at: ending the HIV epidemic: a plan for America (cdc.gov). Available at: https://www.cdc.gov/endhiv/index.html. Accessed October 31, 2022.
9. Branson BM, Handsfield HH, Lampe MA, et al. Revised recommendations for HIV testing of adults, adolescents, and pregnant women in health-care settings. MMWR Recomm Rep (Morb Mortal Wkly Rep) 2006;55. No. RR-14). Available at: https://www.cdc.gov/mmwr/preview/mmwrhtml/rr5514a1.htm.
10. DiNenno EA, Prejean J, Irwin K, et al. Recommendations for HIV screening of gay, bisexual, and other men who have sex with men—United States, 2017. MMWR Morb Mortal Wkly Rep 2017;66:830–2.
11. Hecht J, Sanchez T, Sullivan PS, et al. Increasing access to HIV testing through direct-to-consumer HIV self-test distribution—United States, March 31, 2020-March 30, 2021. Morb Mortal Wkly Rep 2021;70(38):1322–5.
12. Katz DA, Golden MR, Hughes JP, et al. HIV self-testing increases HIV testing frequency in high risk men who have sex with men: a randomized controlled trial. J Acquir Immune Defic Syndr 2018;78(5):505–12.

13. US Food and Drug Administration. FDA approves first over-the-counter home-use rapid HIV test. FDA news release; 2012. Available at: https://www.fda.gov/consumers/consumer-updates/facts-about-home-hiv-testing. Accessed October 31, 2022.

14. Steehler K, Siegler AJ. Bringing HIV self-testing to scale in the United States: a review of challenges, potential solutions, and future opportunities. J Clin Microbiol 2019;57(11):1–12.

15. Pai NP, Vadnais C, Denkinger C, et al. Point-of-care testing for infectious diseases: diversity, complexity, and barriers in low- and middle-income countries. PLoS Med 2012;9(9):e1001306.

16. Herd GC, Musaad SM. Point-of-care testing in rural and remote settings to improve access and improve outcomes: a snapshot of the New Zealand experience. Arch Pathol Lab Med 2021;145:327–35.

17. Valencia J, Lazarus JV, Ceballos FC, et al. Differences in the hepatitis C virus cascade of care and time to initiation of therapy among vulnerable subpopulations using a mobile unit as point-of-care. Liver Int 2022;42:309–19.

18. Makhudu SJ, Kuupiel D, Gwala N, et al. The use of patient self-testing in low- and middle-income countries: a systematic scoping review. Point Care 2019; 18(1):9–16.

19. Bond CS, Hewitt-Taylor J. How people with diabetes integrate self-monitoring of blood glucose into their self-management strategies. Inform Prim Care 2014; 21(2):64–9.

20. Heneghan CJ, Garcia-Alamino JM, Spencer EA, et al. Self-monitoring and self-management of oral anticoagulation. Cochrane Database Syst Rev 2016;7(7): CD003839.

21. Madimenos FC, Gildner TE, Eick GN, et al. Bringing the lab bench to the field: point-of-care testing for enhancing health research and stakeholder engagement in rural/remote, indigenous, and resource-limited contexts. Am J Hum Biol 2022; 34:e23808.

22. Kettler H, White K, Hawkes S. Mapping the landscape of diagnostics for sexually transmitted infections. Geneva: WHO/TDR; 2004.

23. Pai M, Ghiasi M, Pai NP. Point-of-care diagnostic testing in global health: what is the point? Microbe 2015;10(3):103–7.

24. Kost G. Geospatial science and point-of-care testing: creating solutions for population access, emergencies, outbreaks, and disasters. Front Public Health 2019; 7:329.

25. Lau MSY, Gibson GJ, Adrakey H, et al. A mechanistic spatio-temporal framework for modeling individual-to-individual transmission-With an application to the 2014-2015 West Africa Ebola outbreak. PLoS Comput Biol 2017;13:e1005798.

Point-of-Care Testing for Sexually Transmitted Infections

Ashleigh N. Riegler, PhD, Natalie Larsen, MD,
Megan H. Amerson-Brown, PhD*

KEYWORDS

- Sexually transmitted infections • Point-of-care • Diagnostic testing • ASSURED

KEY POINTS

- STI POC tests are available for almost all STIs.
- ASSURED/REASSURED criteria created by the WHO is directing advancements in STI POC testing.
- In high-resource areas, NAAT assays are the preferred POC diagnostic method for most STIs, excluding syphilis, and hepatitis B virus, and hepatitis C virus.
- Limitations to adequate POC testing include cost, ease-of-use, portability, turnaround time, sensitivity, and specificity of assays currently available.
- Future developments in STI diagnostics should focus on the development of POC assays for drug resistance; measuring viral loads; and detecting emerging STIs, such as BV and M genitalium.

INTRODUCTION

Leading public health organizations including the Centers for Disease Control and Prevention (CDC) and World Health Organization (WHO) recognize the importance of sexually transmitted infections (STIs) on the global public health burden and individual sexual and reproductive health.[1–5] STIs are associated with significant morbidity and mortality, with many capable of vertical transmission posing health risks to the fetus.[4] STIs have the highest prevalence in vulnerable populations (men who have sex with men, adolescents, and pregnant women), low-resource, and low-income settings.[6] Concerns for patient autonomy, discomfort, stigma, or loss of privacy often discourage these high-risk and marginalized populations from seeking care for STIs, often leading to a loss of follow-up when infections are identified.[7,8] Many factors

Department of Pathology, The University of Alabama at Birmingham, Marnix E. Heersink School of Medicine, 619 East 19th Street South, WP240J, Birmingham, AL 35249-7331, USA
* Corresponding author.
E-mail address: mamersonbrown@uabmc.edu

Clin Lab Med 43 (2023) 189–207
https://doi.org/10.1016/j.cll.2023.02.006
0272-2712/23/© 2023 Elsevier Inc. All rights reserved.
labmed.theclinics.com

contribute to the persistent infection control and surveillance problems associated with STIs, with the most commonly identified problems being a delay in diagnosis and treatment, and loss to follow-up in which the patient continues to serve as a reservoir.[7,9]

The clinical management of STIs has historically relied on syndromic testing. Many people with active STIs are asymptomatic yet are able to transmit infection. This results in the patient never seeking care or notifying their physician of any problems or histories that would lead to STI testing.[1,9] For most STIs, the likelihood of a correct diagnosis using syndromic management is low. Additionally, syndromic management approaches cannot be effectively used when performing surveillance in a large population. Effective STI prevention and control is dependent on rapid, reliable testing.

In recent years, there has been an increase in recognition of the importance of point-of-care (POC) testing for STIs. According to the CDC, POC testing is defined as rapid testing that is performed close to or near the patient bedside.[10] POC tests have the potential to improve prevention and control of STIs through rapid, same-day diagnosis and initiation of effective therapy, effectually decreasing the need for patient follow-up and reducing the likelihood of transmission and sequelae associated with STIs.[5,11] More than 20 years ago, the WHO developed and published the ASSURED (Affordable, Sensitive, Specific, User-friendly, Rapid and Robust, Equipment-free, and Deliverable) criteria as a way to guide development, standardize testing, and determine whether a POC test addresses the needs for STI diagnosis in low-resource areas.[1,3,4,8] This criterion was designed to combat the universal idea that as the accuracy of a diagnostic test increases, access and affordability of the test decrease. Recently, a renaming of the ASSURED criteria to REASSURED has been proposed with the inclusion of two additional criteria: real-time connectivity and ease of specimen collection.[12]

Since the development of the ASSURED criteria, there have been innovative advances in bacterial, viral, and protozoan STI POC testing and improvements in molecular diagnostic assays making them more accessible to low-resource areas.[5] Despite the plethora of nucleic acid amplification tests (NAAT) that are currently available in high-income, high-resource areas, these tests are often unavailable in low-resource settings including low- and middle-income countries because of cost, funding, personnel, and facility limitations ultimately preventing these populations from benefiting from these assays.[9] This article details examples of currently available POC STI tests, acknowledges tests in currently in development, and identifies areas for improvement and expansion.

TRICHOMONAS VAGINALIS

Trichomonas vaginalis (TV) is the only STI caused by a protozoan. TV is the most common nonviral STI in the United States and can infect men and women. Despite this, TV infections are underdiagnosed because of the high prevalence of asymptomatic infections and the lack of screening guidance. TV infections have been associated with negative outcomes during pregnancy including premature birth and neonatal pneumonia, and have a strong correlation with acquisition and transmission of other STIs.[13–15] Currently, in the United States, the CDC has categorized TV as a neglected parasitic infection.

The historical gold standard for TV diagnostics is direct visualization of trichomonads from a genital swab or urine by microscopy, performed in the laboratory setting or at the bedside. Multiple reports show that this method has poor sensitivity (50%), and requires specialized training.[16–18] Currently, there are five diagnostic tests that are marketed for POC testing: Affirm VPIII (BD Diagnostic Systems, Sparks, MD),

GeneXpert TV (Cepheid, Sunnydale, CA), the Solana HAD Trichomonas (TV) Assay (Quidel Corporation, San Diego, CA), OSOM Trichomonas test (Sekisui Diagnostics, Burlington, MA), and the Kalon TV latex test (Kalon Biological, Surrey, UK). Of these tests currently marketed for POC TV diagnosis, the Affirm VPIII test, Solana HDA Trichomonas Assay, GeneXpert TV Assay, and OSOM Trichomonas test are Food and Drug Administration (FDA)-approved and Clinical Laboratory Improvement Amendments act (CLIA)-waived. Each of these rapid POC tests out-perform microscopy from physician-collected and self-collected samples.[9,18–21]

The Affirm VPIII microbial identification test detects and differentiates between TV, *Candida* sp, and *Gardnerella vaginalis* using nucleic acid capture and complementary DNA probes.[22] Although the ability to test for multiple organisms in a sample provides a clear clinical advantage, multiple studies show that despite the excellent specificity (99%) the VPIII test has varying sensitivities for each target (46%–92%).[21,23,24] Additionally, the Affirm VPIII test is not FDA cleared for use with specimens from men.[24]

The most sensitive assays to detect TV infections are NAAT-based. The GeneXpert TV assay is approved for vaginal, endocervical, and urine samples. The assay provides results within 45 minutes with high sensitivity (97%–99%) and specificity (>99%).[25] Although the assay speed, sensitivity, and specificity meet the ASSURED criteria, the implementation and costs of the GeneXpert system remain too expensive for many low- and middle-income countries.[26] The Solana HDA Trichomonas Assay is a rapid (35 minute) NAAT-based assay approved for vaginal swabs and female urine samples with a high sensitivity (93%–100%) and specificity (>98%).[27,28] The assay is run on the compact, benchtop Solana system and features Quidel's proprietary helicase-dependent amplification (HDA) technology that eliminates the need for a thermocycler. This HDA technology is available for other Solana infectious disease assays ultimately reducing implementation costs.

Unlike the NAAT-based tests for TV, the OSOM trichomonas test and Kalon TV latex tests use antibodies to detect TV-specific antigens that provide a rapid, easy to use bedside diagnosis without the need for additional resources, platforms, or refrigeration to perform the testing, increasing accessibility in low-resource areas and/or field-testing. The OSOM trichomonas test is a single use, low-complexity, dipstick, POC assay to detect TV with a reasonably high sensitivity (83%–90%) and specificity (98.4%–100%).[19] Importantly, compared with the traditional wet mount method, the overall costs for TV diagnosis were significantly decreased with the implementation of the OSOM test.[29] Although the Kalon TV test has also been shown to be effectively used in low-resource settings it has not been cleared for use by the United States or Europe.[16]

GONORRHEA AND CHLAMYDIA

Gonococcal infections are caused by *Neisseria gonorrhoeae* (NG) and most commonly cause urethritis in males and lower or genitourinary tract infections in females. In females, this infection can progress to cause infertility or pelvic inflammatory disease. Surveillance reports have shown an increasing trend of NG infection by 45% since 2016, and that NG infections are associated with an increased risk of acquiring or transmitting other STIs, such as *Chlamydia*, caused by *Chlamydia trachomatis* (CT).[30,31] Although NG and CT differ in infection and pathogenesis, they present with similar signs, symptoms, and potential sequelae. Because of the prevalence and similar clinical presentations, CT and NG are often included on the same POC assays.

The development of assays with reduced complexity and increased sensitivity and specificity has largely replaced nonspecific-based testing, such as leukocyte esterase, especially in high-resource areas. These assays include non-NAAT-based assays, such as BioStar OIA GC (Inverness Medical, Waltham, MA), and NAAT-based assays, such as GeneXpert CT/NG.[28,32] NAAT-based assays are the current recommended assays because of ease of use and high sensitivity and specificity.[28] GeneXpert has two assays, one for NG and one combination test for CT and NG, both of which have been FDA approved for multiple sample types including vaginal, endocervical, pharyngeal, rectal, and urine, with greater than 85% sensitivity and specificity.[33,34] The sensitivity and specificity for extragenital samples do not meet the WHO POC testing requirements.[1,12] Despite the reduced sensitivity associated with some sample types, the GeneXpert assays reduce time to treatment when compared with traditional diagnostic testing making it an optimal assay for high-resource areas.[35–42] The variety of potential sample types that the GeneXpert assays can assess increases the potential testing capabilities in many low-resource areas; however, financial and infrastructure limitations previously discussed often limit the use of the GeneXpert platform in these populations.

In addition to GeneXpert, there are two new NAAT-based POC tests available: Visby Medical Sexual Health Test (Visby Medical, San Jose, CA) and the *binx io* platform (Limited, Boston, MA).[43,44] The Visby Medical Sexual Health Test is a rapid (<30 minutes) single-use diagnostic assay that simultaneously detects CT, NG, and TV with sensitivities and specificities comparable with other NAAT and non-POC test assays (eg, Aptima Combo 2 [Hologic, San Diego, CA] and ProbeTec [Becton Dickinson, Franklin Lakes, NJ]).[28,45] The Visby test received FDA approval and CLIA-waived status in August 2021 and requires no separate instrument or reader, reducing the complication of sample preparation and result interpretation, potentially expanding accessibility for low- and middle-income settings. Currently, the Visby device is only approved for clinician and self-collected vaginal swab samples. Similarly, the *binx io* platform is a polymerase chain reaction (PCR)-based assay for the detection of CT and NG from vaginal swabs and male urine that was CE marked and FDA cleared in 2019, and CLIA-waived in 2021. Like the GeneXpert, the *io* system consists of a fully integrated, benchtop instrument that uses single-use cartridges, and provides a rapid turnaround (30 minutes). When compared with other NAAT based assays, the *io* CT/NG assay had high sensitivity and specificity for vaginal swab samples, but performed at the lower end for sensitivity specificity in male urine samples.[43,46]

The need for mobile, molecular-based CT/NG diagnostic assays, and assays to detect antimicrobial resistance in NG has been recognized and resulted in significant advancements in CT/NG POC testing.[47–49] The quantitative RT cross-priming amplification EasyNAT diagnostic system (Ustar Biotechnologies, Hangzhou, China) includes an all-in-one cartridge and a portable device for amplification and detection of CT and NG. The EasyNAT systems use a cross-priming amplification technique to amplify target sequences at a constant temperature within 80 minutes.[50] This technique reduces the amount of equipment required for analysis, and serves as a novel detection method with the potential for increased access in resource-limited areas.[51] The EasyNAT system will be optimized so that all reagents are stable at ambient air and the assay is expected to obtain CE approval in the near future.[47,49] Similarly, the ResistancePlus GC assay (SpeeDx Pty Ltd, Sydney, Australia), is the first rapid (<60 minutes) commercially available assay that simultaneously detects NG and mutations in *gyrA*, associated with resistance to ciprofloxacin.[52] To address the real-time connectivity criteria of RESSURED, a team at Johns Hopkins University has developed mobile NAAT-based assays: MobiNAAT for CT and PROMPT for NG.[53,54] These assays use a portable, rapid, on-cartridge PCR technology to provide results within 15 minutes. The portability and ease of use with the MobiNAAT and PROMPT assay shows great potential in the future advancements of POC testing for STIs. Although neither of these tests have been approved for clinical use, in clinical trials, they have shown excellent concordance with traditional phenotypic antimicrobial resistance testing and NAAT-based testing.[53,55]

HUMAN IMMUNODEFICIENCY VIRUS (HIV)

Although prevention and early detection are essential for any STI, it is especially important for HIV because of the nature of the infection and potential sequelae. The CDC recommends HIV testing at least once in individuals age 13 to 64, and annual testing for high-risk individuals.[56–58] POC testing for HIV allows for early appropriate initiation of antiretroviral therapy, treatment monitoring, and prevention of opportunistic infections.[59,60] Over the last two decades, numerous easily accessible antibody-based rapid HIV diagnostic tests have been FDA approved, including POC tests and over-the-counter assays, such as the OraQuick In-Home HIV Test (OraSure Technologies, Bethlehem, PA) and the INSTI HIV-1/HIV-2 Antibody Test (Biolytical Laboratories Inc, BC, Canada).[59] Current POC testing options for HIV use a variety of sample types including whole blood, plasma, urine, and oral fluid that allows for improved testing opportunities in patients who prefer less invasive options for sample collection.[59,61] Antibody-based POC diagnostic assays have a high specificity (98%–100%) and sensitivity (>98%) in seroconverted patients. However, in HIV, the window following initial infection and before seroconversion can last up to 12 weeks, during which antibody-based assays cannot detect infection.[60,62] Current, fourth-generation POC tests seek to address the need for earlier diagnosis through the detection of anti-HIV antibodies and the structural viral protein, p24, increasing sensitivity and decreasing the postexposure latency window.[62] Examples of these tests including the Alere HIV Combo Test (Alere Diagnostics, Charlottesville, VA) and the GS HIV Combo Ag/Ab EIA (Bio-Rad Laboratories, Hercules, CA). Despite the shorter window to detection, sensitivity of the assay in patients before seroconversion still remains low (2%–80%).[62]

As with other STI POC tests, NAATs currently have the highest sensitivity and specificity (both >99.9%).[63,64] POC tests to determine HIV viral load are not yet commercially available, requiring samples to be shipped to laboratories for testing.[65,66] Recently, the GeneXpert HIV-1 Quant was evaluated in clinical studies and will likely be added to the growing list of available GeneXpert POC assays.[67] An ideal POC test for HIV viral load would have a limit of detection of less than 1000 copies/mL, give results in less than 1 hour, be easy to use, and inexpensive to perform.[68] The development of POC HIV viral load assays that meet the REASSURED criteria and assays to detect mutations related to drug resistance would be a great advantage to effectively treating HIV infections and preventing transmission.[69]

Additional assays that assist with monitoring HIV infection include monitoring the CD4 T-cell count with less than 200 CD4 cells/mm^3 (normal: 500–1500 cells/mm^3) defining the development of AIDS, and a need for prophylaxis against HIV-associated opportunistic infections.[70] Much like NAATs, traditional CD4 testing requires considerable capital investment and complex training to implement and maintain, impeding their use in resource-limited settings.[71,72] POC CD4 assays, such as PIMA CD4 (Abbott Diagnostics, Charlottesville, VA) and Vitisect CD4 test for advanced HIV (Omega Diagnostics Group, Alva, Scotland) have varying sensitivity (60%–98%), specificity (77%–89%), and diagnostic cutoffs (200–350 cells/

mm³). A study evaluating CD4 assays in Uganda showed acceptable sensitivity and specificity for monitoring disease progression with HIV.[73] Recently, antibody-based combination POC tests that detect HIV and other STIs from a single sample have been developed. These combination assays include HIV, hepatitis B (HBV), hepatitis C (HCV), and syphilis and are also available over the counter.[74–76] The Miriad Rapid HBc/HIV/HCV Antibody Test POU+ (MedMira, Halifax, Nova Scotia) is one such immunochromatographic assay that uses whole blood, plasma, or serum to detect HBc antibodies, HIV1/2 antibodies, and HCV antibodies within 15 minutes. Similarly, the Dual Path Platform (DPP) HIV Syphilis Assay (Chembio Diagnostics Systems, Medford, NY) is an immunochromatographic lateral flow assay for antibodies against syphilis and HIV from a single finger stick. The assay was cleared by the FDA in 2020 and can be stored at room temperature with a shelf-life of 24 months making it ideal for clinics, emergency departments, and field-testing.[77] The development of these assays focuses on screening high-risk populations for multiple STIs on using one sample on one assay.[78]

With all HIV POC tests, counseling, screening strategies, and follow-up confirmatory testing is necessary and should be performed based on local epidemiology and individual risk factors of the relevant patient population. Screening strategies using multiplex assays should be implemented based on local epidemiology of infection and individual risk factors of the patient.[78] Confirmatory tests are almost never POC, because they require a higher specificity or different methods than what is currently available for POC.[60,62,79] Regardless, the benefits of HIV POC testing outweigh the complications as a useful and practical tool to screen high-risk patients and provide a rapid preliminary diagnosis.[79] The development of quantitative HIV POC tests, POC assays to detect mutations related to HIV drug resistance, and further multiplex POC tests that include HIV would be a great advantage to effectively treat HIV infections and prevent transmission.[69]

SYPHILIS

Syphilis is an infection caused by *Treponema pallidum* (TP) and is categorized based on disease pathology and progression: primary (chancre), secondary (maculopapular rash), latent (asymptomatic), and tertiary (any organ can be affected). There are approximately 6 million new cases of syphilis each year, with a 52% increase from 2016 in the United States alone.[30] POC tests currently available have low specificity (<90%), leading to overtreatment. Consequently, these tests are underused for screening purposes, especially pregnant women where it is essential for preventing congenital syphilis.[3] Differentiation between past and present syphilis infection requires multiple tests, with the most sensitive reporting a high false positivity rate and the most specific tests unable to differentiate previous and active infection.[80]

Currently, all available POC diagnostic tests for syphilis rely on the detection of antibodies against the organism (antitreponemal [AT]) or against the products of cellular damage that occurs during infection (nontreponemal [NT]). Antibody-based POC tests for syphilis use immunochromatographic methods and is performed on whole blood, plasma, or serum, providing a result within 30 minutes.[81] POC NT tests are temperature stable, easy to perform, and require minimal instrumentation.[82] These tests include Alere Determine syphilis TP and SD Bioline Syphilis (Abbott Diagnostics, Abbott Park, IL), Syphicheck (Qualpro Diagnostics, Goa, India), and Visitect Syphilis (Omega Diagnostics Ltd, Scotland, UK). The most common NT test type is the rapid plasma reagin test for anticardiolipin (reagin) antibodies. NT tests can result in false-positive results because of production of antireagin antibodies in various nonsyphilis conditions, such as lupus or malaria. False-negative results can occur because of excess antibody overloading the test antigen (termed the prozone effect).[3] In contrast, AT antibody tests have a high sensitivity but cannot distinguish between active and past infection.[3] Available AT tests have similar sensitivity (96%–100%) and specificity (84%– 99%).[83–87] Newer AT assays, such as the BioPoint TP-IgA (Nanjing BioPoint Diagnostics, Nanjing, China), detect TP-specific IgA antibodies that are more sensitive and specific than traditional IgM or IgG detection during active infection.[87]

The most popular syphilis POC assays consist of combination tests that detect AT and NT antibodies, aiding in diagnosing and differentiating active from previous infections. The DPP Syphilis Screen and Confirm Test (Chembio Diagnostics) detects AT and NT antibodies, providing results in less than 15 minutes.[87] The sensitivity and specificity of the NT portion of the DPP does not meet ASSURED criteria, and a recent clinical study showed that DPP did not reduce the number of women overtreated for syphilis.[82] Syphilis testing that can differentiate past and present infection while maintaining high sensitivity may reduce overtreatment and increase screening initiatives.[81] The current POC syphilis testing options cost more than traditional laboratory-based testing. However, the overall cost-benefit associated with reduce infection transmission, and the decrease in disability-adjusted life-years support the value of using and improving syphilis POC testing.[88]

HUMAN PAPILLOMA VIRUS

Human papilloma virus (HPV) includes more than 200 strains, 14 of which are associated with STIs and increased risk for developing cervical cancer.[89] Most HPV testing is performed in high-complexity laboratories, uses highly trained personnel, and has slow turnaround times, and therefore is not sustainable in low-resource areas.[90] In 2020 the WHO launched a global strategy for the elimination of HPV-related cervical cancer, to advance the development and evaluation of HPV screening and treatment approaches.[91,92] There are currently no POC HPV assays that meet the WHO ASSURED criteria. However, two assays are currently available: the Truenat HPV-HR assay (Molbio, Goa, India) and the GeneXpert HPV assay, which indicate the realization of a clinical need for POC HPV testing. Truenat is a portable chip-based test that consists of a sample-processing device and a reverse transcriptase (RT)-PCR analyzer that detects high-risk HPV strains 16, 18, 31, and 45 in cervical samples in less than 1 hour with high sensitivity (86%–99%) and specificity (97%–99%).[93] The Truenat is rechargeable with an 8-hour battery life increasing potential for diagnosis in low-resource areas. The GeneXpert assay detects HPV 16, 18, and 45 using the Xpert RT-PCR cartridge technology.[94] In clinical studies, the GeneXpert had a 90% correlation with traditional testing.[94,95] The sensitivity and specificity of the GeneXpert varied based on the strain of HPV, self- or clinician-collection of sample, overall viral load in the sample, and the cervical intraepithelial neoplasia grade, with increasing specificity as the grade increased.[94,95] With limited POC options available, there is considerable opportunity for improvement in new cost-effective technology and assays that include additional high-risk strains, and improved turnaround times for HPV POC diagnosis.

HERPES SIMPLEX VIRUS

Herpes simplex virus 1 and 2 (HSV-1/2) is one of the most common STIs, with an estimated 12% of the US population being positive for HSV-2 antibodies.[96] HSV-1/2 is a noncurable STI with asymptomatic latency and risk of reactivation. HSV-1/2 presentation is often atypical or subclinical and diagnosis often relies on the presentation of lesions. As with other STIs, the rapid and effective diagnosis of HSV can drastically reduce transmission because of effective treatment and counseling.[97] Currently, the detection of live virus or nucleic acids from lesions is the preferred diagnostic method but relies on symptomatic presentation for adequate sample collection and diagnosis.

Antibody-based POC HSV testing is performed for large population surveillance on samples from asymptomatic patients to determine exposure and infection status. Various lateral-flow assays to detect anti-HSV antibodies are available with high sensitivity (>80%) and specificity (>90%); however, the only commercially available FDA-approved microfluidic antibody-based HSV POC test is the HSV-2 UniGold (Trinity Biotech Plc, Bray, Ireland).[98] This assay uses a portable device to detect HSV-2 gG2 antibodies in approximately 15 minutes.[98] In seroconverted patients, HSV serology is highly sensitive (85%–100%) and specific (97%–100%) when compared with traditional immunoblot testing for HSV-1/2.[97,98] Serology testing can indicate a chronic infection, but it can miss a primary infection, and cannot determine the cause of genital lesions. Therefore, viral detection methods (NAAT, antigen, culture) are needed to diagnose acute infections.[99]

Currently the NAAT-based AmpliVue HSV 1 + 2 and Solana HSV 1 + 2/VZV (Quidel) are the only POC assays available that are performed on swabs from mucosal and genital lesions. The Solana assay is able to differentiate lesions caused by varicella-zoster virus, HSV-1, or HSV-2 with a high sensitivity (91%–100%) and specificity (94%–98%).[98] With the limited number of POC HSV tests available, there is a need to expand and improve these assays to detect and differentiate HSV-1/2 in acute and chronic infection.

BACTERIAL VAGINOSIS

Bacterial vaginosis (BV) is a polymicrobial infection caused by dysregulation of the vaginal microbiome. Although BV is not traditionally considered an STI, epidemiologic and microbiologic studies suggest that sexual transmission is essential to the development of BV.[2,100,101] Historically, BV has been diagnosed at the bedside using Amsel criteria: visual attributes (color and consistency) of the vaginal discharge, presence of amines (measured by whiff test), vaginal pH, and microscopic detection of clue cells in vaginal fluid.[102] Amsel criteria has a low sensitivity and specificity; and vaginal microbial dysregulation can occur without these visible signs or symptoms, resulting in an increased risk of STI acquisition, and preterm birth.[2,103,104] Sensitive and specific POC testing for BV allows for appropriate initiation of therapy, and counseling.[105]

Currently available POC tests for BV detect nonspecific antigens, bacterial species that are correlated with BV but not causative, or vaginal environmental changes. As such, they perform better than traditional syndromic testing yet maintain a low sensitivity and specificity. These tests include OSOM BV Blue Test (Sekisui Diagnostics), which detects sialidase produced by *G vaginalis*, and FemExam pH and Amines Test-Card (Litmus Concepts, Santa Clara, CA), which detects abnormal vaginal pH and amines in vaginal secretions and identifies nonspecific antigens or vaginal environment alterations associated with BV. Likewise, assays to detect BV-associated vaginal inflammation (eg, increased interleukin-1β and IP-10) are currently in development. Although nonspecific for BV, preliminary studies show that this detection of vaginal inflammation has increased sensitivity when compared with Amsel criteria, 77% and 19%, respectively.[103] Detection of vaginal inflammation before the development of more severe BV symptoms may decrease time to diagnosis, initiation of treatment, and incidence of transmission.

Direct detection of BV-associated organisms is more specific than detection of vaginal inflammation biomarkers. The colorimetric BD Affirm VPIII directly detects *G vaginalis*, TV, and *Candida* spp through DNA hybridization technology.[101,106–108] Like the Affirm VPIII, the GeneXpert MVP assay was recently granted 501(k) clearance, and also differentiates BV from TV and *Candida* infections.[109] Utility of the GeneXpert MVP is disputed because it only detects *Atopobium* spp, BV-associated bacterium 2, and *Megasphaera* spp for BV diagnosis, without consideration for the overall bacterial community or other BV-associated organisms, such as *G vaginalis* and *Mycoplasma genitalium*.[110,111] *M genitalium* is an emerging STI that has been recognized as a cause of vaginal inflammation and potential contributor to the development of BV.[104,112–114] Currently, there are no POC tests for the detection of *M genitalium*. The development of rapid POC testing for BV and vaginitis is important for effective STI screening and decreasing pregnancy complications that can arise because of microbiome dysregulation and vaginal inflammation.

SEXUALLY TRANSMITTED INFECTION AT-HOME, SELF-TESTING

At-home, self-testing for STIs provide patients with privacy, confidentiality, convenience, and speed that traditional testing and POCs cannot provide. Additionally, at-home self-testing reduces barriers to health care access and burden on medical systems and personnel that already face staffing shortages. Popularity of at-home test kits has grown since the beginning of the COVID-19 pandemic, and many public health departments and hospital systems now partner with at-home STI testing companies to increase access to STI testing while limiting the burden on clinical staff.[115] Such companies as Binx Health, Inc (Boston, MA), CVS Health (Woonsocket, RI), Everlywell (Austin, TX), and LetsGetChecked (New York, NY) provide sample collection kits and prepaid shipping materials addressed to CLIA-certified and CAP-accredited laboratories for testing.[116,117] Patients follow the package instructions to self-collect urine or swab samples, ship samples with provided materials to the partner laboratory, and receive results less than a week after samples are received by the laboratory. Testing kits are available for HIV, chlamydia, gonorrhea, syphilis, and hepatitis. For those kits provided through a partnership with health departments, positive STI test results are accompanied with connections to in-person follow-up with a health care professional.

Since their introduction nearly a decade ago, multiple reviews have indicated that the availability of STI self-testing has expanded the potential for testing populations with limited access to in-person physician care, and for syphilis and HIV, with similar reliability as traditional POC tests.[118,119] Because of this expanded potential for testing and patient autonomy, in 2019, the WHO issued a report advocating for STI self-testing and proposing adaptions to the established STI testing methods.[120] Soon after this report, the COVID-19 pandemic limited access to in-person clinical STI testing, and laboratories began evaluating the accuracy and reliability of off-label at-home specimen self-collection for STI POC tests, resulting in the implementation of protocol adaptions for tests that were typically performed on physician-collected samples.[121] The increase in demand for at-home STI testing and self-sampling has facilitated the collection and review of implementation-and-use data for these at-home methods, addressing the benefits and issues throughout the United Kingdom and United States.[121,122] At-home testing introduces many of the same risks as traditional, non-POC STI testing, such as lack of follow-up treatment or care. Emphasizing the attrition between testing and follow-up care, reviews of patients who use pharmacy-based infectious disease testing suggest that only 30% to 40% of patients using these services notify a primary care provider.[123,124] Additionally, at home and self-testing for STIs limit community and public health surveillance data; increase the likelihood of unintended, unnecessary, or incorrect use, which subsequently increase the return of incorrect test results; and limit connection to necessary risk counseling or partner notification. Few FDA-approved, CLIA-waived at-home tests are available in which collection and testing are performed at home. These tests have been discussed in previous sections of this article because they related to specific STIs.

THE FUTURE OF SEXUALLY TRANSMITTED INFECTION POINT-OF-CARE TESTING

Incorporating POC testing for STIs into the clinical setting enables clinicians to provide a definitive diagnosis and initiate appropriate treatment, all within the same visit. Some POC testing even allows for implementation of large, on-site community screening in high-risk populations.[1] However, important inhibiting factors for the use of many POC tests for STIs exist: cost; available resources; and regulatory agencies, such as the FDA, WHO, and CLIA, which determine who is qualified to perform the test and whether a test meets quality standards.[27,28] Low sensitivity and specificity of current STI POC tests prove to be additional barriers to clinical implementation.[125] Since the establishment of the ASSURED criteria and the global initiative for STI POC testing, advancements in technology have improved on the sensitivity, specificity, cost, ease of use, sample processing, and result turnaround times (often <15 minutes), yet as discussed throughout, there remains significant room for improvements. Ideal POC STI tests are stored at room temperature, provide results in less than 1 hour, and do not need high-skilled laboratory scientists to perform the test.[126]

Although many new and in-development POC tests for STIs achieve the ASSURED criteria, limitations in current testing exist. NAATs remain the most specific and sensitive STI tests, most of which do not meet ASSURED criteria because of cost and complexity.[127–129] Improvements in NAAT testing should include the development of portable multiplex platforms that do not require a consistent power source. Further reductions in the turnaround times and implementation costs are needed for NAATs. Conversely, immunochromatographic paper-based assays, which are cheap and easy to use, have revolutionized POC testing in developing countries. However, these assays often have less than optimal sensitivities and/or specificity for STI/s, especially when the microbial burden is low.[1,9] Importantly, improvements in all STI POC assays should consider the limitations that exist in the areas or populations where STI prevalence is high, such as the lack of financial means or infrastructural resources in developing countries.

Given the documented increase and growing concern for antimicrobial resistance in STIs, such as NG and HIV, it is paramount that new POC tests be developed to detect resistance to first-line antimicrobial therapy. Potential effects of these combination detection-resistance POC tests include improved patient outcomes, reduced transmission after initiation of treatment, and ultimately reduction of the emergence of antimicrobial resistance in STIs that currently poses a serious health risk.

In addition to detecting antimicrobial resistance, POC tests for STIs are in need of improved detection in nonstandard STI disease presentation or nonstandard sample types, such as those collected from extragenital infections. Expansions in approved sample types that POC tests can screen increases the detection, ultimately reducing the potential damage or transmission related to STI infections. STIs frequently cause extragenital infections including the mouth, throat, and rectum, yet most STI POC tests are not approved for extragenital specimens. This limits the utility of the POC assays and neglects the needs of patients, often in marginalized groups, that experience these nonstandard presentations. Adding to this, most POC STI tests currently available do not include the option for self-collected samples. Self-collection promotes patient autonomy and empowers individuals to take control of their health care. Likewise, it also encourages providers to complete STI screening by eliminating additional time associated with clinician collection.[130–134] Self-collection of specimens with appropriate instruction has been an effective method for specimen collection with accurate results and has shown to increase uptake of screening for STIs in vulnerable populations. POC tests for STIs that allow for expanded sample-type screening including extragenital and self-collected samples have potential to increase the detection and treatment of otherwise damaging, transmissible STIs.

Importantly, considerations for the needs or perceptions of patients and providers, and the clinic workflow, and available resources must guide future advancements in POC testing for STIs.[1,28] The goal of all advancements in POC testing for STIs is to facilitate increased use of POC assays by the physicians; improve patient satisfaction; and increase clinical diagnostic compliance, accuracy, and treatment of STIs. POC testing, even with lower than optimal sensitivity and specificity, can significantly improve treatment and infection prevention efforts by reducing patient attrition between sample collection treatment initiation when compared with traditional methods of syndromic-based testing.[9,11,135] These improvements can be expanded as advancements in STI POC testing options continue to be made.

CLINICS CARE POINTS

- STI POC tests are available for almost all STIs.
- ASSURED/REASSURED criteria created by the WHO is directing advancements in STI POC testing.
- In high-resource areas, NAAT assays are the preferred POC diagnostic method for most STIs, excluding syphilis, and hepatitis B virus, and hepatitis C virus.
- Limitations to adequate POC testing include cost, ease-of-use, portability, turnaround time, sensitivity, and specificity of assays currently available.
- Future developments in STI diagnostics should focus on the development of POC assays for drug resistance; measuring viral loads; and detecting emerging STIs, such as BV and *M genitalium*.

DISCLOSURE

Training and support for A.N. Riegler was provided by NIAID, United States T32AI007051. The authors declare that this article was prepared in the absence of any commercial or financial relationships that could be construed as a potential conflict of interest.

REFERENCES

1. Toskin I, Blondeel K, Peeling RW, et al. Advancing point of care diagnostics for the control and prevention of STIs: the way forward. Sex Transm Infect 2017; 93(S4):S81–8.
2. Unemo M, Bradshaw CS, Hocking JS, et al. Sexually transmitted infections: challenges ahead. Lancet Infect Dis 2017;17(8):e235–79.

3. Sexually Transmitted Diseases Diagnostics Initiative & UNICEF/UNDP/World Bank/WHO, Special Programme for Research and Training in Tropical Diseases. (2006). The use of rapid syphilis tests, World Health Organization; Geneva, Switzerland. https://apps.who.int/iris/handle/10665/43590

4. WHO. UNICEF/UNDP/World bank/WHO special program for research and Training in tropical diseases. Mapping the landscape of diagnostics for sexually transmitted infections. Geneva, Switzerland: World Health Organisation; 2004.

5. Adamson PC, Loeffelholz MJ, Klausner JD. Point-of-care testing for sexually transmitted infections: a review of recent developments. Arch Pathol Lab Med 2020;144(11):1344–51.

6. Unemo M. Accurate, rapid, point-of-care tests for sexually transmitted infections. Lancet Infect Dis 2021;21(5):584–6.

7. Lee ASD, Cody SL. The stigma of sexually transmitted infections. Nurs Clin North Am 2020;55(3):295–305.

8. World Health Organization UNAIDS. United Nations Children's Fund (UNICEF). (2010). Towards universal access: scaling up priority HIV/AIDS interventions in the health sector: progress. In: report. Geneva, Switzerland: World Health Organization; 2010. https://apps.who.int/iris/handle/10665/44443.

9. Gaydos C, Hardick J. Point of care diagnostics for sexually transmitted infections: perspectives and advances. Expert Rev Anti Infect Ther 2014;12(6): 657–72.

10. Prevention CfDCa. Test complexities. 2018. Available at: https://www.cdc.gov/clia/test-complexities.html. Accessed October 3, 2022.

11. Rönn MM, Menzies NA, Gift TL, et al. Potential for point-of-care tests to reduce chlamydia-associated burden in the United States: a mathematical modeling analysis. Clin Infect Dis 2020;70(9):1816–23.

12. Land KJ, Boeras DI, Chen X-S, et al. REASSURED diagnostics to inform disease control strategies, strengthen health systems and improve patient outcomes. Nature Microbiology 2019;4(1):46–54.

13. Mavedzenge SN, Pol BV, Cheng H, et al. Epidemiological synergy of Trichomonas vaginalis and HIV in Zimbabwean and South African women. Sex Transm Dis 2010;37(7):460–6.

14. McClelland RS, Sangaré L, Hassan WM, et al. Infection with Trichomonas vaginalis increases the risk of HIV-1 acquisition. J Infect Dis 2007;195(5):698–702.

15. Li RT, Lin HC, Chung CH, et al. Trichomonas infection in pregnant women: a nationwide cohort study. Parasitol Res 2022;121(7):1973–81.

16. Hobbs MM, Seña AC. Modern diagnosis of Trichomonas vaginalis infection. Sex Transm Infect 2013;89(6):434–8.

17. Madico G, Quinn TC, Rompalo A, et al. Diagnosis of Trichomonas vaginalis infection by PCR using vaginal swab samples. J Clin Microbiol 1998;36(11): 3205–10.

18. Huppert JS, Mortensen JE, Reed JL, et al. Rapid antigen testing compares favorably with transcription-mediated amplification assay for the detection of Trichomonas vaginalis in young women. Clin Infect Dis 2007;45(2):194–8.

19. Hawash Y. Ease of use and validity testing of a point-of-care fast test for parasitic vaginosis self-diagnosis. Trop Biomed 2021;38(4):491–8.

20. Wendel KA, Erbelding EJ, Gaydos CA, et al. Trichomonas vaginalis polymerase chain reaction compared with standard diagnostic and therapeutic protocols for detection and treatment of vaginal trichomoniasis. Clin Infect Dis 2002;35(5): 576–80.

21. Brown HL, Fuller DD, Jasper LT, et al. Clinical evaluation of affirm VPIII in the detection and identification of *Trichomonas vaginalis*, *Gardnerella vaginalis*, and *Candida* species in vaginitis/vaginosis. Infect Dis Obstet Gynecol 2004; 12(1):17–21.
22. Gazi H, Degerli K, Kurt O, et al. Use of DNA hybridization test for diagnosing bacterial vaginosis in women with symptoms suggestive of infection. Apmis 2006;114(11):784–7.
23. Levi AW, Harigopal M, Hui P, et al. Comparison of Affirm VPIII and Papanicolaou tests in the detection of infectious vaginitis. Am J Clin Pathol 2011;135(3):442–7.
24. Dessai F, Nyirenda M, Sebitloane M, et al. Diagnostic evaluation of the BD Affirm VPIII assay as a point-of-care test for the diagnosis of bacterial vaginosis, trichomoniasis and candidiasis. Int J STD AIDS 2020;31(4):303–11.
25. Schwebke JR, Gaydos CA, Davis T, et al. Clinical evaluation of the cepheid Xpert TV assay for detection of trichomonas vaginalis with prospectively collected specimens from men and women. J Clin Microbiol 2018;56(2).
26. Martin K, Roper T, Vera JH. Point-of-care testing for sexually transmitted infections in low- and middle-income countries: a scoping review protocol. JBI Evid Synth 2021;19(1):155–62.
27. Gaydos CA, Klausner JD, Pai NP, et al. Rapid and point-of-care tests for the diagnosis of *Trichomonas vaginalis* in women and men. Sex Transm Infect 2017;93(S4):S31–5.
28. Gaydos CA, Manabe YC, Melendez JH. A narrative review of where we are with point-of-care sexually transmitted infection testing in the United States. Sex Transm Dis 2021;48(8s):S71–s77.
29. Campbell L, Woods V, Lloyd T, et al. Evaluation of the OSOM Trichomonas rapid test versus wet preparation examination for detection of *Trichomonas vaginalis* vaginitis in specimens from women with a low prevalence of infection. J Clin Microbiol 2008;46(10):3467–9.
30. Division of STD Prevention, National Center for HIV, Viral Hepatitis, STD, and TB Prevention, Centers for Disease Control and Prevention (August 22, 2022). "Sexually Transmitted Disease Surveillance 2020." Available at: https://www. cdc.gov/std/statistics/2020/default.htm. Accessed September, 08, 2022.
31. Pettifor A, Walsh J, Wilkins V, et al. How effective is syndromic management of STDs?: a review of current studies. Sex Transm Dis 2000;27(7):371–85.
32. Samarawickrama A, Alexander S, Ison C. A laboratory-based evaluation of the Biostar optical immunoassay point-of-care test for diagnosing *Neisseria gonorrhoeae* infection. J Med Microbiol 2011;60(12):1779–81.
33. Gaydos CA, Van Der Pol B, Jett-Goheen M, et al. Performance of the cepheid CT/NG Xpert rapid PCR test for detection of *Chlamydia trachomatis* and *Neisseria gonorrhoeae*. J Clin Microbiol 2013;51(6):1666–72.
34. Cepheid, GeneXpert CT/NG package insert, Cepheid, 2019, Sunnyvale, CA, USA.
35. Wingrove I, Mcowan A, Nwokolo N, et al. Diagnostics within the clinic to test for gonorrhoea and chlamydia reduces the time to treatment: a service evaluation. Sex Transm Infect 2014;90:474.
36. Hesse EA, Widdice LE, Patterson-Rose SA, et al. Feasibility and acceptability of point-of-care testing for sexually transmissible infections among men and women in mobile van settings. Sex Health 2015;12 1:71–3.
37. Bristow CC, Mathelier P, Ocheretina O, et al. *Chlamydia trachomatis*, *Neisseria gonorrhoeae*, and *Trichomonas vaginalis* screening and treatment of pregnant women in Port-au-Prince, Haiti. Int J STD AIDS 2017;28(11):1130–4.

38. Mandlik E, Plaha K, Jones R, et al. P101 Cutting the time to treatment of *Chlamydia trachomatis* (CT) and *Neisseria gonorrhoeae* (NG) with near-patient molecular diagnostics: the utility of the cepheid GeneXpert system. Sex Transm Infect 2017;93(Suppl 1):A49.44–9.

39. Bell SFE, Coffey L, Debattista J, et al. Peer-delivered point-of-care testing for *Chlamydia trachomatis* and *Neisseria gonorrhoeae* within an urban community setting: a cross-sectional analysis. Sex Health 2020;17(4):359.

40. Whitlock GG, Gibbons DC, Longford N, et al. Rapid testing and treatment for sexually transmitted infections improve patient care and yield public health benefits. Int J STD AIDS 2018;29(5):474–82.

41. Harding-Esch EM, Nori AV, Hegazi A, et al. Impact of deploying multiple point-of-care tests with a 'sample first' approach on a sexual health clinical care pathway. A service evaluation. Sex Transm Infect 2017;93(6):424–9.

42. Rivard KR, Dumkow LE, Draper HM, et al. Impact of rapid diagnostic testing for chlamydia and gonorrhea on appropriate antimicrobial utilization in the emergency department. Diagn Microbiol Infect Dis 2017;87(2):175–9.

43. Van Der Pol B, Gaydos CA. A profile of the Binx health *io* molecular point-of-care test for chlamydia and gonorrhea in women and men. Expert Rev Mol Diagn 2021;21(9):861–8.

44. Van Der Pol B, Taylor SN, Mena L, et al. Evaluation of the performance of a point-of-care test for chlamydia and gonorrhea. JAMA Netw Open 2020;3(5):e204819.

45. Morris SR, Bristow CC, Wierzbicki MR, et al. Performance of a single-use, rapid, point-of-care PCR device for the detection of *Neisseria gonorrhoeae*, *Chlamydia trachomatis*, and *Trichomonas vaginalis*: a cross-sectional study. Lancet Infect Dis 2021;21(5):668–76.

46. Harding-Esch EM, Cousins EC, Chow SLC, et al. A 30-min nucleic acid amplification point-of-care test for genital *Chlamydia trachomatis* infection in women: a prospective, multi-center study of diagnostic accuracy. EBioMedicine 2018;28:120–7.

47. Murtagh MM. *The Point-of-Care Diagnostic Landscape for Sexually Transmitted Infections (STIs)*. Geneva, Switzerland: The Murtagh Group LLC; 2019. https://cdn.who.int/media/docs/default-source/hrp/pocts/diagnostic-landscape-for-stis-2019.pdf?sfvrsn=52ae633f_9.

48. Wi T, Lahra MM, Ndowa F, et al. Antimicrobial resistance in *Neisseria gonorrhoeae*: global surveillance and a call for international collaborative action. PLoS Med 2017;14(7):e1002344.

49. Thakur SD, Levett PN, Horsman GB, et al. High levels of susceptibility to new and older antibiotics in *Neisseria gonorrhoeae* isolates from Saskatchewan (2003–15): time to consider point-of-care or molecular testing for precision treatment? J Antimicrob Chemother 2018;73(1):118–25.

50. Xu G, Hu L, Zhong H, et al. Cross priming amplification: mechanism and optimization for isothermal DNA amplification. Sci Rep 2012;2(1):246.

51. Yu B, An Y, Xu G, et al. Detection of *Chlamydia trachomatis* and *Neisseria gonorrhoeae* based on cross-priming amplification. Lett Appl Microbiol 2016;62(5):399–403.

52. Ebeyan S, Windsor M, Bordin A, et al. Evaluation of the ResistancePlus GC (beta) assay: a commercial diagnostic test for the direct detection of ciprofloxacin susceptibility or resistance in *Neisseria gonorrhoeae*. J Antimicrob Chemother 2019;74(7):1820–4.

53. Trick AY, Melendez JH, Chen FE, et al. A portable magnetofluidic platform for detecting sexually transmitted infections and antimicrobial susceptibility. Sci Transl Med 2021;13(593).

54. Shin DJ, Athamanolap P, Chen L, et al. Mobile nucleic acid amplification testing (mobiNAAT) for *Chlamydia trachomatis* screening in hospital emergency department settings. Sci Rep 2017;7:4495.

55. Chen L, Shin DJ, Zheng S, et al. Direct-qPCR assay for coupled identification and antimicrobial susceptibility testing of *Neisseria gonorrhoeae*. ACS Infect Dis 2018;4(9):1377–84.

56. Eu B, Roth N, Stoové M, et al. Rapid HIV testing increases the rate of HIV detection in men who have sex with men: using rapid HIV testing in a primary care clinic. Sex Health 2014;11(1):89–90.

57. Ciaranello AL, Park J-E, Ramirez-Avila L, et al. Early infant HIV-1 diagnosis programs in resource-limited settings: opportunities for improved outcomes and more cost-effective interventions. BMC Med 2011;9(1):59.

58. Reid S, Fidler SJ, Cooke GS. Tracking the progress of HIV: the impact of point-of-care tests on antiretroviral therapy. Clin Epidemiol 2013;387–96.

59. Arora DR, Maheshwari M, Arora B. Rapid point-of-care testing for detection of HIV and clinical monitoring. ISRN AIDS 2013;2013:1–5.

60. Pottie K, Medu O, Welch V, et al. Effect of rapid HIV testing on HIV incidence and services in populations at high risk for HIV exposure: an equity-focused systematic review. BMJ Open 2014;4(12):e006859.

61. Minichiello A, Swab M, Chongo M, et al. HIV point-of-care testing in Canadian settings: a scoping review. Front Public Health 2017;5:76.

62. Chetty V, Moodley D, Chuturgoon A. Evaluation of a 4th generation rapid HIV test for earlier and reliable detection of HIV infection in pregnancy. J Clin Virol 2012;54(2):180–4.

63. Stekler JD, Swenson PD, Coombs RW, et al. HIV testing in a high-incidence population: is antibody testing alone good enough? Clin Infect Dis 2009;49(3):444–53.

64. Tan WS, Chow EPF, Fairley CK, et al. Sensitivity of HIV rapid tests compared with fourth-generation enzyme immunoassays or HIV RNA tests. AIDS 2016;30(12):1951–60.

65. Sherman GG, Stevens G, Jones SA, et al. Dried blood spots improve access to HIV diagnosis and care for infants in low-resource settings. JAIDS Journal of Acquired Immune Deficiency Syndromes 2005;38(5):615–7.

66. Defo D, Kouotou EA, Nansseu JR. Failure to return to receive HIV-test results: the Cameroon experience. BMC Res Notes 2017;10(1):309.

67. Manavi K, Hodson J, Masuka S, et al. Correlation between cepheid GeneXpert and Abbott M2000 assays for HIV viral load measurements. Int J STD AIDS 2021;32(5):444–8.

68. Estill J, Egger M, Blaser N, et al. Cost-effectiveness of point-of-care viral load monitoring of antiretroviral therapy in resource-limited settings: mathematical modelling study. Aids 2013;27(9):1483–92.

69. Drain PK, Dorward J, Bender A, et al. Point-of-Care HIV viral load testing: an essential tool for a sustainable global HIV/AIDS response. Clin Microbiol Rev 2019;32(3). e00097-e00018.

70. Vidya Vijayan KK, Karthigeyan KP, Tripathi SP, et al. Pathophysiology of CD4+ T-cell depletion in HIV-1 and HIV-2 infections. Front Immunol 2017;8:580.

71. Kohatsu L, Bolu O, Schmitz ME, et al. Evaluation of specimen types for Pima CD4 point-of-care testing: advantages of fingerstick blood collection into an EDTA microtube. PLoS One 2018;13(8):e0202018.

72. Ndlovu Z, Massaquoi L, Bangwen NE, et al. Diagnostic performance and usability of the VISITECT CD4 semi-quantitative test for advanced HIV disease screening. PLoS One 2020;15(4):e0230453.

73. Namuniina A, Lutwama F, Biribawa VM, et al. Field performance of PIMA point-of-care machine for CD4 enumeration under a mobile HIV counseling and testing program in remote fishing communities of Lake Victoria, Uganda. AIDS Res Hum Retrovir 2019;35(4):382–7.

74. Ceesay A, Lemoine M, Cohen D, et al. Clinical utility of the 'determine HBsAg' point-of-care test for diagnosis of hepatitis B surface antigen in Africa. Expert Rev Mol Diagn 2022;22(5):497–505.

75. Uusküla A, Talu A, Rannap J, et al. Rapid point-of-care (POC) testing for hepatitis C antibodies in a very high prevalence setting: persons injecting drugs in Tallinn, Estonia. J Harm Reduct 2021;18:39–45.

76. Van Den Heuvel A, Smet H, Prat I, et al. Laboratory evaluation of four HIV/syphilis rapid diagnostic tests. BMC Infect Dis 2019;19(1). https://doi.org/10.1186/s12879-018-3567-x.

77. US Food and Drug Administration. (2020). "DPP HIV-Syphilis System." Available at: https://www.fda.gov/vaccines-blood-biologics/blood-blood-products/dpp-hiv-syphilis-system. Accessed October 24, 2022.

78. Pawlotsky J-M. The importance of point-of-care tests for HCV and HBV in the implementation of WHO strategy of viral hepatitis elimination by 2030. Geneva, Switzerland: EASL: International Liver Foundation; 2019.

79. Kagulire SC, Opendi P, Stamper PD, et al. Field evaluation of five rapid diagnostic tests for screening of HIV-1 infections in rural Rakai, Uganda. Int J STD AIDS 2011;22(6):308–9.

80. Satyaputra F, Hendry S, Braddick M, et al. The laboratory diagnosis of syphilis. J Clin Microbiol 2021;59(10):e00100–21.

81. Morshed MG, Singh AE. Recent trends in the serologic diagnosis of syphilis. Clin Vaccine Immunol 2015;22(2):137–47.

82. Constantine NT, Sill AM, Gudesblat E, et al. Assessment of two rapid assays for diagnostic capability to accurately identify infection by *Treponema pallidum*. The Journal of Applied Laboratory Medicine 2017;1(4):346–56.

83. Jafari Y, Peeling RW, Shivkumar S, et al. Are *Treponema pallidum* specific rapid and point-of-care tests for syphilis accurate enough for screening in resource limited settings? Evidence from a meta-analysis. PLoS One 2013;8(2):e54695.

84. Sabidó M, Benzaken AS, de-Andrade-Rodrigues EJ, et al. Rapid point-of-care diagnostic test for syphilis in high-risk populations, Manaus, Brazil. Emerg Infect Dis 2009;15(4):647–9.

85. Diaz T, De Gloria Bonecini Almeida M, Georg I, et al. Evaluation of the determine rapid syphilis TP assay using sera. Clin Vaccine Immunol 2004;11(1):98–101.

86. Mabey D, Peeling RW, Ballard R, et al. Prospective, multi-centre clinic-based evaluation of four rapid diagnostic tests for syphilis. Sex Transm Infect 2006; 82(Suppl 5):v13–6.

87. Pham MD, Wise A, Garcia ML, et al. Improving the coverage and accuracy of syphilis testing: the development of a novel rapid, point-of-care test for confirmatory testing of active syphilis infection and its early evaluation in China and South Africa. EClinicalMedicine 2020;24:100440.

88. Romero CP, Marinho DS, Castro R, et al. Cost-effectiveness analysis of point-of-care rapid testing versus laboratory-based testing for antenatal screening of syphilis in Brazil. Value in Health Regional Issues 2020;23:61–9.
89. Chan CK, Aimagambetova G, Ukybassova T, et al. Human papillomavirus infection and cervical cancer: epidemiology, screening, and vaccination. Review of current perspectives. Journal of Oncology 2019;2019:3257939.
90. Sayed S, Chung M, Temmerman M. Point-of-care HPV molecular diagnostics for a test-and-treat model in high-risk HIV populations. Lancet Global Health 2020; 8(2):e171–2.
91. Global strategy to accelerate the elimination of cervical cancer as a public health problem. Geneva, Switzerland: World Health Organization; 2020.
92. Vallely AJB, Saville M, Badman SG, et al. Point-of-care HPV DNA testing of self-collected specimens and same-day thermal ablation for the early detection and treatment of cervical pre-cancer in women in Papua New Guinea: a prospective, single-arm intervention trial (HPV-STAT). Lancet Global Health 2022;10(9): e1336–46.
93. Hariprasad R, Tulsyan S, Babu R, et al. Evaluation of a chip-based, point-of-care, portable, real-time micro PCR analyzer for the detection of high-risk human papillomavirus in uterine cervix in India. JCO Global Oncology 2020;(6): 1147–54.
94. Mbulawa ZZA, Wilkin TJ, Goeieman B, et al. Xpert human papillomavirus test is a promising cervical cancer screening test for HIV-seropositive women. Papillomavirus Res 2016;2:56–60.
95. Saidu R, Kuhn L, Tergas A, et al. Performance of Xpert HPV on self-collected vaginal samples for cervical cancer screening among women in South Africa. J Low Genit Tract Dis 2021;25(1):15–21.
96. Kreisel KM, Spicknall IH, Gargano JW, et al. Sexually transmitted infections among US women and men: prevalence and incidence estimates, 2018. Sex Transm Dis 2021;48(4):208–14.
97. Philip SS, Ahrens K, Shayevich C, et al. Evaluation of a new point-of-care serologic assay for herpes simplex virus type 2 infection. Clin Infect Dis 2008;47(10): e79–82.
98. Nath P, Kabir MA, Doust SK, et al. Diagnosis of herpes simplex virus: laboratory and point-of-care techniques. Infect Dis Rep 2021;13(2):518–39.
99. Arshad Z, Alturkistani A, Brindley D, et al. Tools for the diagnosis of herpes simplex virus 1/2: systematic review of studies published between 2012 and 2018. JMIR Public Health and Surveillance 2019;5(2):e14216.
100. Kairys N, Garg M. Bacterial Vaginosis. In: StatPearls [Internet]. Treasure Island (FL). StatPearls Publishing; 2022.
101. Muzny CA, Balkus J, Mitchell C, et al. Diagnosis and management of bacterial vaginosis: summary of evidence reviewed for the 2021 centers for disease control and prevention sexually transmitted infections treatment guidelines. Clin Infect Dis 2022;74(Supplement_2):S144–51.
102. Amsel R, Totten PA, Spiegel CA, et al. Nonspecific vaginitis. Diagnostic criteria and microbial and epidemiologic associations. Am J Med 1983;74(1):14–22.
103. Kairu A, Masson L, Passmore J-AS, et al. Rapid point-of-care testing for genital tract inflammatory cytokine biomarkers to diagnose asymptomatic sexually transmitted infections and bacterial vaginosis in women: cost estimation and budget impact analysis. Sex Transm Dis 2022;49(3):237–43.
104. Shipitsyna E, Khusnutdinova T, Budilovskaya O, et al. Bacterial vaginosis-associated vaginal microbiota is an age-independent risk factor for *Chlamydia*

trachomatis, Mycoplasma genitalium and *Trichomonas vaginalis* infections in low-risk women, St. Petersburg, Russia. Eur J Clin Microbiol Infect Dis 2020; 39(7):1221–30.

105. Pai N, Ghiasi M, Pai M. Point-of-care diagnostic testing in global health: what is the point? Microbe 2015;10:103–7.

106. Bradshaw CS, Morton AN, Garland SM, et al. Evaluation of a point-of-care test, BVBlue, and clinical and laboratory criteria for diagnosis of bacterial vaginosis. J Clin Microbiol 2005;43(3):1304–8.

107. West B, Morison L, Schim van der Loeff M, et al. Evaluation of a new rapid diagnostic kit (FemExam) for bacterial vaginosis in patients with vaginal discharge syndrome in the Gambia. Sex Transm Dis 2003;30(6):483–9.

108. Pappas S, Makrilakis K, Anyfantis I, et al. Clinical evaluation of affirm VP III in the detection and identification of bacterial vaginosis. J Chemother 2008;20(6): 764–5.

109. FDA. "510(k) SUBSTANTIAL EQUIVALENCE DETERMINATION DECISION SUMMARY ASSAY AND INSTRUMENT." Available at: https://www.accessdata.fda. gov/cdrh_docs/reviews/K212213.pdf. Accessed October 18, 202.

110. Anton L, Ferguson B, Friedman ES, et al. *Gardnerella vaginalis* alters cervicovaginal epithelial cell function through microbe-specific immune responses. Microbiome 2022;10(1):119.

111. Nye MB, Harris AB, Pherson AJ, et al. Prevalence of *Mycoplasma genitalium* infection in women with bacterial vaginosis. BMC Wom Health 2020;20(1):62.

112. Gaydos C, Maldeis NE, Hardick A, et al. *Mycoplasma genitalium* as a contributor to the multiple etiologies of cervicitis in women attending sexually transmitted disease clinics. Sex Transm Dis 2009;36(10):598–606.

113. Lokken EM, Balkus JE, Kiarie J, et al. Association of recent bacterial vaginosis with acquisition of *Mycoplasma genitalium*. Am J Epidemiol 2017;186(2): 194–201.

114. Seña AC, Lee JY, Schwebke J, et al. A silent epidemic: the prevalence, incidence and persistence of *Mycoplasma genitalium* among young, asymptomatic high-risk women in the United States. Clin Infect Dis 2018;67(1):73–9.

115. Carnevale C, Richards P, Cohall R, et al. At-home testing for sexually transmitted infections during the COVID-19 pandemic. Sex Transm Dis 2021;48(1):e11–4.

116. Department APH. STI prevention and control STD/HIV home testing. 2021. Available at: https://www.alabamapublichealth.gov/std/home-testing.html. Accessed 2/3/2023.

117. Francis MS, Ashley K, Bruno T. Results of comprehensive sexually transmitted disease testing utilizing an at-home kit over one year [27J]. Obstet Gynecol 2019;133:114S–5S.

118. Turner KME, Looker KJ, Syred J, et al. Online testing for sexually transmitted infections: a whole systems approach to predicting value. PLoS One 2019;14(2): e0212420.

119. Smit PW, van der Vlis T, Mabey D, et al. The development and validation of dried blood spots for external quality assurance of syphilis serology. BMC Infect Dis 2013;13:102.

120. WHO consolidated guideline on self-care interventions for health: sexual and reproductive health and rights. Geneva: World Health Organization; 2019.

121. Kersh EN, Shukla M, Raphael BH, et al. At-home specimen self-collection and self-testing for sexually transmitted infection screening demand accelerated by the COVID-19 pandemic: a review of laboratory implementation issues. J Clin Microbiol 2021;59(11). e02646-e02620.

122. Sumray K, Lloyd KC, Estcourt CS, et al. Access to, usage and clinical outcomes of, online postal sexually transmitted infection services: a scoping review. Sex Transm Infect 2022;98(7):528–35.
123. Klepser DG, Klepser ME, Dering-Anderson AM, et al. Community pharmacist-physician collaborative streptococcal pharyngitis management program. J Am Pharm Assoc (2003) 2016;56(3):323–9.e321.
124. Klepser ME, Klepser DG, Dering-Anderson AM, et al. Effectiveness of a pharmacist-physician collaborative program to manage influenza-like illness. J Am Pharm Assoc (2003) 2016;56(1):14–21.
125. Hsieh Y-H, Gaydos CA, Hogan MT, et al. What qualities are most important to making a point of care test desirable for clinicians and others offering sexually transmitted infection testing? PLoS One 2011;6(4):e19263.
126. Peeling RW, Holmes KK, Mabey D, et al. Rapid tests for sexually transmitted infections (STIs): the way forward. Sex Transm Infect 2006;82(Suppl 5):v1–6.
127. Herbst De Cortina S, Bristow CC, Joseph Davey D, et al. A systematic review of point of care testing for *Chlamydia trachomatis*, *Neisseria gonorrhoeae*, and *Trichomonas vaginalis*. Infect Dis Obstet Gynecol 2016;2016:1–17.
128. Watchirs Smith LA, Hillman R, Ward J, et al. Point-of-care tests for the diagnosis of *Neisseria gonorrhoeae* infection: a systematic review of operational and performance characteristics. Sex Transm Infect 2013;89(4):320–6.
129. Gaydos CA, Melendez JH. Point-by-point progress: gonorrhea point of care tests. Expert Rev Mol Diagn 2020;20(8):803–13.
130. Lunny C, Taylor D, Hoang L, et al. Self-collected versus clinician-collected sampling for chlamydia and gonorrhea screening: a systemic review and meta-analysis. PLoS One 2015;10(7):e0132776.
131. Chapman KS, Gadkowski LB, Janelle J, et al. Automated sexual history and self-collection of extragenital chlamydia and gonorrhea improve detection of bacterial sexually transmitted infections in people with HIV. AIDS Patient Care STDS 2022;36(S2):104–10.
132. Chow EPF, Bradshaw CS, Williamson DA, et al. Changing from clinician-collected to self-collected throat swabs for oropharyngeal gonorrhea and chlamydia screening among men who have sex with men. J Clin Microbiol 2020;58(9).
133. Khan Z, Bhargava A, Mittal P, et al. Evaluation of reliability of self-collected vaginal swabs over physician-collected samples for diagnosis of bacterial vaginosis, candidiasis and trichomoniasis, in a resource-limited setting: a cross-sectional study in India. BMJ Open 2019;9(8):e025013.
134. Ogale Y, Yeh PT, Kennedy CE, et al. Self-collection of samples as an additional approach to deliver testing services for sexually transmitted infections: a systematic review and meta-analysis. BMJ Glob Health 2019;4(2):e001349.
135. Van Der Pol B. Making the most of point-of-care testing for sexually transmitted diseases. Clin Infect Dis 2020;70(9):1824–5.

Point-of-Care Testing for the Diagnosis of Fungal Infections

Current Testing Applications and Potential for the Future

Paul M. Luethy, PhD, D(ABMM)

KEYWORDS:

- Fungal diagnostics • *Aspergillus* • Galactomannan • Lateral flow assay • NAAT
- LAMP

KEY POINTS

- Fungal infections are increasing due to the increased number of individuals with immunocompromised or immunosuppressed conditions.
- Traditional fungal diagnostics require lengthy incubations or processes and are often insensitive with varying specificity.
- Rapid and easy-to-perform lateral flow assays for fungal antigens have been developed and could be useful in the point-of-care setting.
- The advancement of loop-mediated isothermal amplification methods will lead to the development of molecular fungal point-of-care testing in the near future.

INTRODUCTION

In comparison to bacteria and viruses, fungi represent a small slice of the infectious pie, yet fungal diseases cause more than an estimated 1.6 million deaths annually.[1] Typical fungal infections in the immunocompetent individual are limited to superficial infections of hair, nails, and skin. Invasive fungal infections, however, are beginning to increase as a result of increased numbers of immunosuppressed and/or immunocompromised individuals due to the development and use of novel immunomodulating therapies.[1,2] In addition, the warming climate has led to the spread of fungi that were once thought geographically or seasonally limited, raising concerns for an increase in infections by these agents.[3] The high morbidity and mortality of invasive infections warrants the development of rapid and easily accessible diagnostic tools.

Department of Pathology, University of Maryland School of Medicine, 22 South Greene Street, Room N2E31, Baltimore, MD 21201, USA
E-mail address: pluethy@som.umaryland.edu

Clin Lab Med 43 (2023) 209–220
https://doi.org/10.1016/j.cll.2023.02.005
0272-2712/23/© 2023 Elsevier Inc. All rights reserved.
labmed.theclinics.com

However, unlike bacteria and viruses, the development of novel fungal diagnostics that could be used in the point-of-care (POC) setting is often overlooked.

The current gold-standard methodologies for the diagnosis of fungal infections requires the procurement of either a superficial (hair clippings, piece of nail, a skin scraping) or an invasive (tissue, body fluid, respiratory) specimen for culture and/or pathologic evaluation. Unfortunately, both of these techniques take an extended amount of time, are often insensitive, and require extensive training. The detection of fungal biomarkers by lateral flow technology has been incorporated into the diagnostic algorithm. These assays offer a simplified and often more rapid approach to diagnosis than culture or histopathology, although performance of the assay may require more complex procedures than found in a POC setting at this time.

Recent developments in fungal diagnostics have resulted in the creation of nucleic acid amplification tests (NAAT) (such as polymerase chain reaction [PCR]) for the detection of filamentous fungi directly from specimens. In particular, assays have focused on the detection of *Aspergillus* species and the Mucorales, with some commercial assays available with limited regulatory approval.[4] Further, multiplexed NAATs have been developed to quickly identify yeast grown in blood culture bottles, which can result in rapid changes to appropriate antifungal therapy.[5] Unfortunately, no POC molecular testing for fungi is available at this time.

This review summarizes lateral flow and molecular testing for the detection of fungi while commenting on the potential for use in the POC setting.

DISCUSSION
Lateral Flow Assays

Cryptococcal lateral flow assays

Perhaps the assay type with the most promise for POC testing are lateral flow assays (LFAs). LFAs are simple to use tests in which a liquid sample is applied to a paper-based test platform.[6] Many LFAs for use in the POC setting have been developed for bacterial and viral targets; however, relatively few LFAs are available for fungal diagnosis in the laboratory setting (**Table 1**). Likely the most well-known of the LFAs for fungal detection is the cryptococcal antigen LFA or CrAg. Performance of the CrAg assay within the laboratory from blood and cerebrospinal fluid (CSF) specimens has demonstrated fantastic sensitivity and specificity for the diagnosis of cryptococcosis.[7] Although this assay has not been approved for POC testing, the ability to be performed with limited facilities at room temperature and the low cost per test strip increases its POC potential, especially in resource-limited settings.[8] As such, several studies have been conducted to evaluate the feasibility of POC testing using the CrAg LFA.[8–10] These studies found that the CrAg LFA remained sensitive and specific when performed in resource-limited settings, even with delicate samples such as CSF[8] and when performed by lay persons in rural Africa.[10] However, some limitations to POC testing are still apparent, such as the need for sample volumes larger than finger prick blood.[9]

Further advancements have been made in the detection of CrAg as new LFAs are developed. One of the limitations of CrAg testing is the need to perform titers upon initial detection. Although not the most complex testing, the creation of a dilution series represents a potential pitfall to the POC environment. To simplify the process, 2 semiquantitative LFAs for the detection of CrAg have been developed for testing of serum and CSF specimens.[11,12] Although more data are needed to correlate the new semiquantitative measures with traditional titers and patient outcomes, the high sensitivity and specificity of the newer LFAs combined with the semiquantitation may lead to a rapid adoption in the POC environment.

Table 1
Commercially available lateral flow tests for the detection of fungal infections

Assay Name	Organism	Specimen	Specific Target	FDA or CE Approval	Reference
Immy Cryptococcal Antigen LFA	Cryptococcus species	Serum, CSF	Cryptococcus capsular polysaccharide antigens	FDA and CE	Rick et al,[10] 2017
BIOSYNEX CryptoPS	Cryptococcus species	Serum, plasma, whole blood, CSF	Cryptococcus capsular polysaccharide antigens	CE	Ocansey et al,[14] 2022
Immy CrAg SQ	Cryptococcus species	Serum	Cryptococcus capsular polysaccharide antigens	Neither	Ocansey et al,[14] 2022
Immy sōna Coccidioides Antibody LFA	Coccidioides species	Serum, CSF	Anti-Coccidioides IgM and IgG	FDA (serum)	Caillot et al,[19] 1997
MiraVista Histoplasma Urine Antigen LFA	Histoplasma species	Urine	Histoplasma galactomannan	CE	Jenks & Hoenigl,[18] 2020
Immy sōna Aspergillus GM LFA	Aspergillus species	Serum, BALF	Aspergillus galactomannan	CE	Wiederhold et al,[23] 2009
OLM Diagnostics Aspergillus-specific LFD	Aspergillus species	Serum, BALF	Aspergillus extracellular glycoprotein	FDA and CE	Almeida-Paes et al,[26] 2022

A second advancement is the development of CrAg LFAs that are compatible with additional samples that are easy to obtain. As such, a study has been performed that assessed the detection of the cryptococcal polysaccharide capsule glucuronoxylomannan by an LFA in serum, plasma, and urine samples.[13] The study showed promising results for the interchangeability of serum and plasma, potentially allowing for shared specimens for CrAg testing and CD4 cell counts following HIV diagnosis. In addition, the study found promising results with the LFA and urine specimens, demonstrating a potential portability to noninvasive samples found typically in the POC setting.

Aspergillus lateral flow assays

The use of LFAs for the detection of fungi besides *Cryptococcus* species has remained largely under development. Assays have been developed for the diagnosis of histoplasmosis,[14,15] coccidioidomycosis,[16] *Pneumocystis* pneumonia,[17] and aspergillosis.[18] Currently, only the LFA for the detection of *Coccidioides* species immunoglobulin G (IgG) and IgM in serum has received Food and Drug Administration (FDA) approval, with the assay demonstrating a good negative predictive value due to its high specificity albeit lower positive predictive value and sensitivity.[16] *Pneumocystis* LFAs fall on the opposite side of the spectrum as a promising yet still developing research-based method,[17] and *Histoplasma* detection by LFA falls somewhere in the middle with both LFAs having achieved a CE-mark for the detection of antigen in urine with high sensitivity and specificity.[14,15]

The early detection of invasive aspergillosis is important, as the rapid adjustment to appropriate therapy can improve rates of survival.[19] Current diagnostic algorithms for the detection of disease include culture, histopathology, as well as enzyme-linked immunosorbent assay (ELISA) for galactomannan (a polysaccharide that primarily exists in the cell wall of *Aspergillus* species) in serum and bronchoalveolar lavage fluid (BALF). However, galactomannan (GM) ELISA testing is largely limited to reference laboratories due to the special equipment, setup, and time required to perform this assay. Furthermore, reports of false-positive results due to contamination through dietary consumption of GM-containing foods, cross-reactivity with other fungi, and reactivity with prior formulations of piperacillin-tazobactam have limited the GM ELISA utility.[20] As such, the development of lateral flow tests for the detection of *Aspergillus* in a variety of specimens has been highly studied.[21,22] One such lateral flow device (LFD) uses monoclonal antibodies to detect an extracellular glycoprotein secreted by *Aspergillus* species during active growth.[23,24] Early studies of the Aspergillus-specific LFD with serum specimens found earlier times to positivity in a guinea pig model when compared with the standard biomarkers GM and β-D glucan.[23] Additional work has focused on migrating the GM ELISA to an LFA.[21] Both of these assays have been refined and distilled into commercial products.

Two lateral flow tests have received CE-marking for the detection of *Aspergillus* in BALF and serum: the sōna *Aspergillus* GM LFA and the *Aspergillus*-specific LFD (AspLFD).[18,21] Both diagnostic tests have been studied extensively for their sensitivity, specificity, and utility in patients with hematologic malignancies and limited studies in those with solid organ transplants and patients in intensive care.[18,21,25–29] Overall sensitivity and specificity of the GM LFA for differentiating a probable or proven case of invasive aspergillosis compared with a negative case was found to be 77% and 81%, respectively,[25] although these values increased to 83% to 89% sensitivity and 87% to 88% specificity when only patients with hematological malignancy were studied.[21] Interestingly, the GM LFA exhibited the lowest sensitivity and specificity in solid organ transplant recipients, although the results are limited to one single-center study.[21] Surprisingly, the sensitivity and specify of the GM LFA was higher in intensive care unit (ICU) patients (61% and 80%, respectively) than in those with solid organ transplants. Further studies are needed to confirm this trend, however, as both the solid organ transplant and ICU results are from individual single-center studies.

The AspLFD exhibited similar characteristics to the GM LFA in hematological malignancy patients[18,29] in cases of proven invasive pulmonary aspergillosis. Sensitivity of the LFD decreased in proven and probable cases, although specificity remained the same as the LFA. Both the GM LFA and AspLFD have been tested for the detection of Aspergillus in nonneutropenic patients.[26,28] Samples in the GM LFA study were included from patients with chronic pulmonary aspergillosis, aspergilloma, invasive aspergillosis, and COVID-19–associated pulmonary aspergillosis,[26] whereas the AspLFD was tested for those with chronic pulmonary aspergillosis, subacute invasive pulmonary aspergillosis, and aspergilloma.[28] Each study compared the assays versus the GM ELISA used in clinical care; the GM LFA was found to have a lower sensitivity than the ELISA but a higher specificity when testing serum samples, whereas the AspLFD was found to have similar sensitivity and higher specificity depending on the ELISA cut-off value. Further, the AspLFD was tested in BALF in comparison to the GM ELISA and was found to have lower sensitivity and specificity than the GM ELISA assay.

One concern with lateral flow tests is a potential to misread the results of the assay. A weak positive test line may occur due to poor sample collection, an error in sample processing, the hook effect, or due to a low amount of overall analyte present in the sample.[6] One way to assist in the reading of these faintly positive results is to use a reader instrument. Reader instruments are commonly used for antigen tests such as human immunodeficiency virus antibody differentiation testing.[30] The use of a reader instrument increases the likelihood of appropriately reading the GM LFA and AspLFD results.[29] The increase in diagnostic performance with the use of a reader instrument may still depend on the patient population, however, as studies of BALF in solid organ transplant and ICU patients found that specificity benefited greatly with the reader, whereas sensitivity was dependent on using specific cut-offs.[21,25] For instance, increasing the cut-off from 1.0 Optical Density Index (ODI) to 2.0 ODI in solid organ transplant patients resulted in an increase of specificity from 42% to 83%, and a change of 1.0 ODI to 1.5 ODI resulted in an increase of specificity from 75% to 83% in ICU patients.

The ultimate goal of an Aspergillus LFA or LFD would be utilization in the POC environment. Unfortunately, neither commercial assay has achieved that distinction at this time, likely due to several cumbersome processing steps. However, just as the AspLFD and LFA were developed and tested over time, so too are LFA assays that may help to push the testing into the POC space. Using urine as the specimen of choice, a new LFD has been developed that uses a galactofuranose-specific anti-Aspergillus fumigatus monoclonal antibody to rapidly detect fungal antigen.[31] A recent study using urine samples from patients undergoing evaluation for fungal infection found an overall sensitivity of 80% and specificity of 92%. Similar to the studies of the GM LFA and AspLFD, sensitivity was highest in patients with cancer and lowest in those without cancer. Although preliminary, this new LFD represents a promising advancement for the diagnosis of invasive aspergillosis in the POC environment.

Lateral flow assay clinics care points

- Lateral flow tests are simple to perform and are under development for many fungal species. However, these are precluded from POC testing often due to multiple sample processing steps.

- Population studies are necessary to determine the correct patients for testing, such as shown in the case for *Aspergillus* GM LFA and *Asp*LFD in hematological malignancy patients but not solid organ transplant patients.

Molecular Testing

Rapid molecular diagnostics have transformed the practice of clinical microbiology both in the high complexity laboratory and in the POC space. In comparison to antigen-based assays (including LFAs and LFDs), molecular diagnostic assays boast of improved sensitivity and specificity,[32] even at the POC level. The traditional flow of molecular diagnostics has been reengineered to allow for rapid testing on small and simple devices. Examples of POC molecular assays that have been developed include group A *Streptococcus*, [33] SARS-CoV-2,[34] Influenza A/B and RSV,[35–37] and sexually transmitted infections.[38] Development of new molecular POC tests is ongoing, with particular interest in isothermal technology that requires minimal instrumentation, such as loop-mediated isothermal amplification (LAMP).[39] Although molecular diagnostics serve as the likely future for POC testing, no POC molecular assays for the detection of fungal infections are available at this time. However, it is important to note that few molecular fungal tests have been FDA approved at all. One test, the T2Candida Panel (T2 Biosystems, Lexington, MA, USA), has been FDA approved for detection of *Candida* species directly from a blood draw and is described later. High complexity molecular testing for fungal infections is a broad area of study, and multistep PCR tests have been developed for a number of fungal pathogens, including *Aspergillus*, *Pneumocystis jirovecii*, *Candida* species, and the Mucorales.[40–42] Other fungi, such as the dermatophytes, have also been targeted for detection by molecular assays.[43] Optimal use of molecular assays for the detection of fungal infections is often when combined with serologic tests for β-D-glucan and/or GM. Next-generation sequencing assays are the latest development in high complexity molecular testing, and studies have shown it is capable of the detection of pulmonary invasive fungal infections,[44] although the cost and complexity are prohibitively high for day-to-day laboratory diagnosis.

Recent developments in FDA-approved molecular fungal testing in the moderate and high complexity laboratory has focused on a sample-to-answer approach. These assays allow for random access testing of multiple tests from different specimens on one instrument and contain multiple probes to allow for the detection of several pathogens at once. However, these assays first require culture to amplify organism concentration and serve to detect positive cultures rather than the pathogen directly from a specimen. Examples include the BioFire Blood Culture Identification 2 panel, which can detect the emerging pathogen *Candida auris*,[45] and the GenMark Dx ePlex system, which can simultaneously detect 15 fungal targets including common *Candida* species, both *Cryptococcus gattii* and *Cryptococcus neoformans*, as well as *Fusarium* species and *Rhodotorula* species.[5]

Multiplexed molecular assays such as those described earlier succeed in providing a rapid, sensitive, and specific test for fungal pathogens. However, to move closer to POC testing, these assays must be able to be performed outside of clinical laboratory and with specimens that do not require incubation. Further, as blood cultures are negative in approximately 50% of invasive candidiasis cases,[46] a culture-based molecular assay for fungi suffers from the lower sensitivity of culture even though the sensitivity of the molecular test is very high. One approach to solve this is through the use of T2 magnetic resonance.[22,46,47] Sample collection requires simply a K_2 EDTA blood collection tube and placing it upon the dedicated instrument for sample processing and target detection. Evaluation of the assay showed the ability to detect

Cryptococcus albicans/Cryptococcus tropicalis, *Cryptococcus parapsilosis*, and *Cryptococcus krusei/Cryptococcus glabrata* with a sensitivity of 91.1% within 4 to 5 hours,[48] and organisms could be detected even following antifungal therapy.[49] Although promising, there are a few characteristics that preclude the T2 magnetic resonance method from being used in the POC environment. First, the assay requires a large and expensive instrument that is unwieldy for urgent care clinics and similar environments. Second, the assay, although more rapid than a blood culture, requires several hours before producing a result. Lastly, initial studies have shown an up to 9% invalid rate,[46] which would lead to multiple specimen draws and repeated testing.

Molecular clinics care points

- Molecular techniques increase sensitivity and specificity of testing. However, current fungal molecular diagnostics are required to be performed in high complexity laboratories.
- Multiplexed sample-to-answer testing provides rapid results in an easy-to-perform test. However, these assays often require a positive culture to increase assays sensitivity.
- Isothermal amplification techniques such as LAMP will likely become adapted to the POC space due to few equipment requirements and rapid turn-around-time. Assays for fungal targets are under development.

WHAT MIGHT THE FUTURE HOLD FOR FUNGAL POINT-OF-CARE TESTING?

Despite the lack of currently approved and available POC assays for the detection of invasive fungal infections, there remains a high need for the development of rapid, inexpensive, and accessible tests. The recent announcement by the World Health Organization (WHO) lists *C neoformans*, *A fumigatus*, *C auris*, and *C albicans* as critical priority fungal pathogens for the development of new assays and public health measures.[50] As such, the continued development of tests using lateral flow or LAMP technology with easily obtainable specimens will be instrumental in addressing this global need. For example, imagine genus-specific lateral flow tests that can detect invasive fungal infections directly from the blood or urine with little pretreatment or processing steps. Such a urine-based test is under development for the detection of *Aspergillus*, *Histoplasma*, and *Cryptococcus* antigens.[13,14,31,51] Many more molds, such as *Fusarium*, *Scedosporium*, *Coccidioides*, and *Lomentospora* species, which are defined as high- and medium-priority fungal pathogens by the WHO,[50] represent new targets for novel LFA and LFD development. *Pneumocystis*, which was classified as medium priority, has seen initial development of a lateral flow immunoassay that showed promising results.[17]

Molecular testing through rapid testing methods such as LAMP offer another path to POC fungal testing. The isothermal nature and limited technology required for LAMP testing are characteristics that make it ideal for both the small clinic and resource-limited settings.[39,52] Although still under development, LAMP has been used to detect the veterinary pathogens *Trichophyton mentagrophytes* and *Microsporum canis*,[53] which are the most common fungal species isolated from cats and dogs. The LAMP assay demonstrated high sensitivity and specificity from hair samples when compared with a quantitative multiplex PCR. With this success, one can envision further LAMP assays for the detection of human dermatophytes using hair and skin specimens.

LAMP assays have also been prototyped for the detection of *P jirovecii*[54] and *A fumigatus*.[55] In both studies, the LAMP assay was compared with a traditional PCR assay and found to have similar performance characteristics while also allowing for rapid detection (under 17 minutes for the *Pneumocystis* assay and 75 minutes for the *Aspergillus* assay). However, further study and development is needed for these assays, as the *Pneumocystis* assay could not differentiate between colonization and probable infection, whereas the *Aspergillus* assay required an extensive (20 minutes) DNA preparation process that would be cumbersome in the POC setting.

SUMMARY

Although POC testing for fungal infections is still squarely on the horizon, advancements in molecular and lateral flow technologies will rapidly accelerate the timeline for assay creation and adoption. Future developments will likely include the use of handhold devices, such as smart phones, that will aid in the ease of use, portability, and interpretation of the lateral flow and molecular techniques, especially in resource-limited environments.[56] As fungal infections continue to increase and garner increased international recognition, so too will the need for easily accessible POC fungal diagnostics.

DISCLOSURE

P.M. Luethy has performed consulting work with bioMerieux.

REFERENCES

1. Almeida F, Rodrigues ML, Coelho C. The still underestimated problem of fungal diseases worldwide. Front Microbiol 2019;10:214. https://doi.org/10.3389/fmicb. 2019.00214.
2. Seagle EE, Williams SL, Chiller TM. Recent trends in the epidemiology of fungal infections. Infect Dis Clin North Am 2021;35(2):237–60. https://doi.org/10.1016/j. idc.2021.03.001.
3. Nnadi NE, Carter DA. Climate change and the emergence of fungal pathogens. Plos Pathog 2021;17(4):e1009503. https://doi.org/10.1371/journal.ppat.1009503.
4. Zhang SX, Babady NE, Hanson KE, et al. Recognition of diagnostic gaps for laboratory diagnosis of fungal diseases: expert opinion from the fungal diagnostics laboratories consortium (FDLC). J Clin Microbiol 2021;59(7):e0178420. https:// doi.org/10.1128/JCM.01784-20.
5. Zhang SX, Carroll KC, Lewis S, et al. Multicenter evaluation of a PCR-based digital microfluidics and electrochemical detection system for the rapid identification of 15 fungal pathogens directly from positive blood cultures. J Clin Microbiol 2020;58(5). 020966-e2119.
6. Koczula KM, Gallotta A. Lateral flow assays. Essays Biochem 2016;60(1):111–20. https://doi.org/10.1042/EBC20150012.
7. Boulware DR, Rolfes MA, Rajasingham R, et al. Multisite validation of cryptococcal antigen lateral flow assay and quantification by laser thermal contrast. Emerg Infect Dis 2014;20(1):45–53. https://doi.org/10.3201/eid2001.130906.
8. Kabanda T, Siedner MJ, Klausner JD, et al. Point-of-care diagnosis and prognostication of cryptococcal meningitis with the cryptococcal antigen lateral flow assay on cerebrospinal fluid. Clin Infect Dis 2014;58(1):113–6. https://doi.org/ 10.1093/cid/cit641.
9. WAKE RM, JARVIS JN, HARRISON TS, et al. Point of care cryptococcal antigen screening: pipetting finger-prick blood improves performance of immunomycologics lateral flow assay. J Acquir Immune Defic Syndr 2018;78(5):574–8. https://doi.org/10.1097/QAI.0000000000001721.

10. Rick F, Niyibizi AA, Shroufi A, et al. Cryptococcal antigen screening by lay cadres using a rapid test at the point of care: a feasibility study in rural Lesotho. PLoS One 2017;12(9):e0183656. https://doi.org/10.1371/journal.pone.0183656.

11. Skipper C, Tadeo K, Martyn E, et al. Evaluation of serum cryptococcal antigen testing using two novel semiquantitative lateral flow assays in persons with cryptococcal antigenemia. J Clin Microbiol 2020;58(4). https://doi.org/10.1128/JCM.02046-19. 020466-e2119.

12. Tadeo KK, Nimwesiga A, Kwizera R, et al. Evaluation of the diagnostic performance of a semiquantitative cryptococcal antigen point-of-care assay among HIV-infected persons with cryptococcal meningitis. J Clin Microbiol 2021;59(8): e0086021. https://doi.org/10.1128/JCM.00860-21.

13. Jarvis JN, Percival A, Bauman S, et al. Evaluation of a novel point-of-care cryptococcal antigen test on serum, plasma, and urine from patients with HIV-associated cryptococcal meningitis. Clin Infect Dis 2011;53(10):1019–23. https://doi.org/10.1093/cid/cir613.

14. Ocansey BK, Otoo B, Asamoah I, et al. Cryptococcal and Histoplasma antigen screening among people with human immunodeficiency virus in Ghana and comparative analysis of OIDx Histoplasma lateral flow assay and IMMY Histoplasma enzyme immunoassay. Open Forum Infect Dis 2022;9(7):ofac277. https://doi.org/10.1093/ofid/ofac277.

15. Cáceres DH, Gómez BL, Tobón AM, et al. Evaluation of a Histoplasma antigen lateral flow assay for the rapid diagnosis of progressive disseminated histoplasmosis in Colombian patients with AIDS. Mycoses 2020;63(2):139–44. https://doi.org/10.1111/myc.13023.

16. Donovan FM, Ramadan FA, Khan SA, et al. Comparison of a novel rapid lateral flow assay to enzyme immunoassay results for early diagnosis of coccidioidomycosis. Clin Infect Dis 2021;73(9):e2746–53. https://doi.org/10.1093/cid/ciaa1205.

17. Tomás AL, de Almeida MP, Cardoso F, et al. Development of a gold nanoparticle-based lateral-flow immunoassay for Pneumocystis pneumonia serological diagnosis at point-of-care. Front Microbiol 2019;10:2917. https://doi.org/10.3389/fmicb.2019.02917.

18. Jenks JD, Hoenigl M. Point-of-care diagnostics for invasive aspergillosis: nearing the finish line. Expert Rev Mol Diagn 2020;20(10):1009–17. https://doi.org/10.1080/14737159.2020.1820864.

19. Caillot D, Casasnovas O, Bernard A, et al. Improved management of invasive pulmonary aspergillosis in neutropenic patients using early thoracic computed tomographic scan and surgery. J Clin Oncol 1997;15(1):139–47. https://doi.org/10.1200/JCO.1997.15.1.139.

20. Lim ZY, Ho AYL, Devereux S, et al. False positive results of galactomannan ELISA assay in haemato-oncology patients: a single centre experience. J Infect 2007; 55(2):201–2. https://doi.org/10.1016/j.jinf.2006.11.015.

21. Jenks JD, Miceli MH, Prattes J, et al. The Aspergillus lateral flow assay for the diagnosis of invasive aspergillosis: an update. Curr Fungal Infect Rep 2020; 14(4):378–83. https://doi.org/10.1007/s12281-020-00409-z.

22. Patterson TF, Donnelly JP. New concepts in diagnostics for invasive mycoses: non-culture-based methodologies. J Fungi (Basel) 2019;5(1):E9. https://doi.org/10.3390/jof5010009.

23. Wiederhold NP, Thornton CR, Najvar LK, et al. Comparison of lateral flow technology and galactomannan and (1->3)-beta-D-glucan assays for detection of invasive pulmonary aspergillosis. Clin Vaccin Immunol 2009;16(12):1844–6. https://doi.org/10.1128/CVI.00268-09.

24. Zhang L, Guo Z, Xie S, et al. The performance of galactomannan in combination with 1,3-β-D-glucan or aspergillus-lateral flow device for the diagnosis of invasive aspergillosis: evidences from 13 studies. Diagn Microbiol Infect Dis 2019;93(1):44–53. https://doi.org/10.1016/j.diagmicrobio.2018.08.005.

25. Jenks JD, Prattes J, Frank J, et al. Performance of the bronchoalveolar lavage fluid Aspergillus galactomannan lateral flow assay with cube reader for diagnosis of invasive pulmonary aspergillosis: a multicenter cohort study. Clin Infect Dis 2021;73(7):e1737–44. https://doi.org/10.1093/cid/ciaa1281.

26. Almeida-Paes R, Almeida M de A, de Macedo PM, et al. Performance of two commercial assays for the detection of serum Aspergillus galactomannan in non-neutropenic patients. J Fungi (Basel) 2022;8(7):741. https://doi.org/10.3390/jof8070741.

27. Heldt S, Prattes J, Eigl S, et al. Diagnosis of invasive aspergillosis in hematological malignancy patients: performance of cytokines, Asp LFD, and Aspergillus PCR in same day blood and bronchoalveolar lavage samples. J Infect 2018;77(3):235–41. https://doi.org/10.1016/j.jinf.2018.05.001.

28. Takazono T, Ito Y, Tashiro M, et al. Evaluation of aspergillus-specific lateral-flow device test using serum and bronchoalveolar lavage fluid for diagnosis of chronic pulmonary aspergillosis. J Clin Microbiol 2019;57(5). https://doi.org/10.1128/JCM.00095-19. 000955-e119.

29. Mercier T, Dunbar A, de Kort E, et al. Lateral flow assays for diagnosing invasive pulmonary aspergillosis in adult hematology patients: a comparative multicenter study. Med Mycol 2020;58(4):444–52. https://doi.org/10.1093/mmy/myz079.

30. Montesinos I, Eykmans J, Delforge ML. Evaluation of the Bio-Rad Geenius HIV-1/2 test as a confirmatory assay. J Clin Virol 2014;60(4):399–401. https://doi.org/10.1016/j.jcv.2014.04.025.

31. Marr KA, Datta K, Mehta S, et al. Urine antigen detection as an aid to diagnose invasive aspergillosis. Clin Infect Dis 2018;67(11):1705–11. https://doi.org/10.1093/cid/ciy326.

32. Schmitz JE, Stratton CW, Persing DH, et al. Forty years of molecular diagnostics for infectious diseases. J Clin Microbiol 2022;19:e0244621. https://doi.org/10.1128/jcm.02446-21.

33. Wang F, Tian Y, Chen L, et al. Accurate detection of Streptococcus pyogenes at the point of care using the cobas liat strep A nucleic acid test. Clin Pediatr (Phila) 2017;56(12):1128–34. https://doi.org/10.1177/0009922816684602.

34. Lee J, Song JU. Diagnostic accuracy of the Cepheid Xpert Xpress and the Abbott ID NOW assay for rapid detection of SARS-CoV-2: a systematic review and meta-analysis. J Med Virol 2021;93(7):4523–31. https://doi.org/10.1002/jmv.26994.

35. Yin N, Van Nuffelen M, Bartiaux M, et al. Clinical impact of the rapid molecular detection of RSV and influenza A and B viruses in the emergency department. PLoS One 2022;17(9):e0274222. https://doi.org/10.1371/journal.pone.0274222.

36. Morehouse ZP, Chance N, Ryan GL, et al. A narrative review of nine commercial point of care influenza tests: an overview of methods, benefits, and drawbacks to rapid influenza diagnostic testing. J Osteopath Med 2022. https://doi.org/10.1515/jom-2022-0065.

37. Azar MM, Landry ML. Detection of influenza A and B viruses and respiratory syncytial virus by use of clinical laboratory improvement amendments of 1988 (CLIA)-Waived point-of-care assays: a paradigm shift to molecular tests. J Clin Microbiol 2018;56(7). https://doi.org/10.1128/JCM.00367-18. 003677-e418.

38. Adamson PC, Loeffelholz MJ, Klausner JD. Point-of-Care testing for sexually transmitted infections: a review of recent developments. Arch Pathol Lab Med 2020;144(11):1344–51. https://doi.org/10.5858/arpa.2020-0118-RA.

39. Moehling TJ, Choi G, Dugan LC, et al. LAMP diagnostics at the point-of-care: emerging trends and perspectives for the developer community. Expert Rev Mol Diagn 2021;21(1):43–61. https://doi.org/10.1080/14737159.2021.1873769.

40. White PL, Alanio A, Brown L, et al. An overview of using fungal DNA for the diagnosis of invasive mycoses. Expert Rev Mol Diagn 2022;22(2):169–84. https://doi.org/10.1080/14737159.2022.2037423.

41. Millon L, Caillot D, Berceanu A, et al. Evaluation of serum Mucorales polymerase chain reaction (PCR) for the diagnosis of mucormycoses: the MODIMUCOR prospective trial. Clin Infect Dis 2022;75(5):777–85. https://doi.org/10.1093/cid/ciab1066.

42. Seo H, Kim JY, Son HJ, et al. Diagnostic performance of real-time polymerase chain reaction assay on blood for invasive aspergillosis and mucormycosis. Mycoses 2021;64(12):1554–62. https://doi.org/10.1111/myc.13319.

43. Ross IL, Weldhagen GF, Kidd SE. Detection and identification of dermatophyte fungi in clinical samples using a commercial multiplex tandem PCR assay. Pathology 2020;52(4):473–7. https://doi.org/10.1016/j.pathol.2020.03.002.

44. Wang C, You Z, Fu J, et al. Application of metagenomic next-generation sequencing in the diagnosis of pulmonary invasive fungal disease. Front Cell Infect Microbiol 2022;12:949505. https://doi.org/10.3389/fcimb.2022.949505.

45. Sparks R, Balgahom R, Janto C, et al. Evaluation of the BioFire Blood Culture Identification 2 panel and impact on patient management and antimicrobial stewardship. Pathology 2021;53(7):889–95. https://doi.org/10.1016/j.pathol.2021.02.016.

46. Clancy CJ, Nguyen MH. Diagnosing invasive candidiasis. J Clin Microbiol 2018;56(5):e01909–17. https://doi.org/10.1128/JCM.01909-17.

47. Clancy CJ, Nguyen MH. Non-culture diagnostics for invasive candidiasis: promise and unintended consequences. J Fungi (Basel) 2018;4(1):E27. https://doi.org/10.3390/jof4010027.

48. Mylonakis E, Clancy CJ, Ostrosky-Zeichner L, et al. T2 magnetic resonance assay for the rapid diagnosis of candidemia in whole blood: a clinical trial. Clin Infect Dis 2015;60(6):892–9. https://doi.org/10.1093/cid/ciu959.

49. Clancy CJ, Pappas PG, Vazquez J, et al. Detecting infections rapidly and easily for candidemia trial, Part 2 (DIRECT2): a prospective, multicenter study of the T2Candida panel. Clin Infect Dis 2018;66(11):1678–86. https://doi.org/10.1093/cid/cix1095.

50. Geneva: World Health Organization. WHO fungal priority pathogens list to guide research, development and public health action. 2022. Available at: https://www.who.int/publications-detail-redirect/9789240060241. Accessed October 25, 2022.

51. Abdallah W, Myint T, LaRue R, et al. Diagnosis of histoplasmosis using the MVista Histoplasma galactomannan antigen qualitative lateral flow-based immunoassay: a multicenter study. Open Forum Infect Dis 2021;8(9):ofab454. https://doi.org/10.1093/ofid/ofab454.

52. Hassan MM, Grist LF, Poirier AC, et al. JMM profile: loop-mediated isothermal amplification (LAMP): for the rapid detection of nucleic acid targets in resource-limited settings. J Med Microbiol 2022;71(5). https://doi.org/10.1099/jmm.0.001522.

53. Müs Tak HK, Ünal G, Müs Tak INBA. Detection of Microsporum canis and Tricho-phyton mentagrophytes by loop-mediated isothermal amplification (LAMP) and real-time quantitative PCR (qPCR) methods. Vet Dermatol 2022. https://doi.org/10.1111/vde.13111.

54. Ng WWY, Ho YII, Wong AH, et al. Comparison of PneumID real-time PCR assay with Amplex eazyplex LAMP assay for laboratory diagnosis of Pneumocystis jir-ovecii Pneumonia. Med Mycol 2022;myac043. https://doi.org/10.1093/mmy/myac043.

55. Jiang L, Gu R, Li X, et al. Simple and rapid detection Aspergillus fumigatus by loop-mediated isothermal amplification coupled with lateral flow biosensor assay. J Appl Microbiol 2021;131(5):2351–60. https://doi.org/10.1111/jam.15092.

56. García-Bernalt Diego J, Fernández-Soto P, Márquez-Sánchez S, et al. SMART-LAMP: a smartphone-operated handheld device for real-time colorimetric point-of-care diagnosis of infectious diseases via loop-mediated isothermal amplifica-tion. Biosensors (Basel) 2022;12(6):424. https://doi.org/10.3390/bios12060424.

Hot Topics in Cancer Testing and New Developments

Metaplastic Breast Carcinoma Revisited; Subtypes Determine Outcomes
Comprehensive Pathologic, Clinical, and Molecular Review

Thaer Khoury, MD

KEYWORDS

- Metaplastic carcinoma • Triple-negative breast cancer • Histologic subtype
- Spindle cell lesion • Immunohistochemistry • Immunotherapy • Molecular subtypes
- Diagnostic algorithm

KEY POINTS

- Metaplastic breast carcinoma (MpBC) is a heterogeneous group of tumors that clinically could be divided into low risk and high risk.
- It is important to recognize the different types of MpBC, as the high-risk subtypes have worse clinical outcomes than triple-negative breast cancer.
- Spindle cell lesion of the breast has a wide range of differential diagnoses. It is important for the pathologist to be aware of the MpBC entities and use the herein proposed algorithms to assist in the diagnosis.
- Metaplastic breast carcinoma has less response rate to the traditional chemotherapy (adjuvant or neoadjuvant) than the other types of breast cancer.
- Few options of target therapies and immunotherapy are available for the patients with MpBC.

OVERVIEW

The name origin of metaplasia is from the Greek verb *metaplasein*, which means "change in form." It is the transformation from one differentiated cell type to another differentiated cell type. Metaplastic breast carcinoma (MpBC) is a heterogeneous group of tumors that have only one thing in common. The tumor cells transformed

This article originally appeared in *Surgical Pathology Clinics* Volume 15 Issue 1, March 2022.
Pathology Department, Roswell Park Comprehensive Cancer Center, Elm & Carlton Streets, Buffalo, NY 14263, USA
E-mail address: thaer.khoury@roswellpark.org
Twitter: @KhouryThaer (T.K.)

Clin Lab Med 43 (2023) 221–243
https://doi.org/10.1016/j.cll.2023.03.002
0272-2712/23/© 2023 Elsevier Inc. All rights reserved.

labmed.theclinics.com

from the benign mammary cell (epithelial or myoepithelial) to a cell type with malignant properties such as squamous cell, chondroid cells, and so forth. These tumors have more differences than similarities, including the morphology, the biology, and more importantly the prognosis and therefore the management.

The World Health Organization (WHO) classified these tumors into 5 subtypes: low-grade adenosquamous carcinoma (LGASC), fibromatosis-like metaplastic carcinoma (FLMC), squamous cell carcinoma (SqCC), spindle cell carcinoma (SpCC), and metaplastic carcinoma with heterologous mesenchymal differentiation (MCHMD). When a tumor has mixed components, it is designated as mixed metaplastic carcinoma (MMC).[1] In this review, the following subjects are going to be discussed: the histomorphologic features of each subtype, a proposed approach to spindle cell lesions detected in a core needle biopsy (CNB) with the differential diagnosis and the immunohistochemistry (IHC) workup, the molecular alterations, tumor microenvironment, and up-to-date target therapy and immunotherapy.

PATHOLOGY
Histologic Subtypes

Low-Grade Adenosquamous Carcinoma
The LGASC is an ill-defined tumor with infiltrating borders, composed of a mixture of infiltrating neoplastic glandular and squamous structures, all present in the background of sclerotic or desmoplastic stroma with bland nuclear morphology.[2] The glandular component usually reveals well-developed glandular and tubular formations with minimal, if any, angulation, unlike tubular carcinoma. The squamous component varies from extensive epidermoid growth, syringoma-like differentiation, and isolated small clusters and solid nests.[3] The overall nuclear grade is low with minimal, if any, mitotic figures. Aggregates of lymphocytes located within or at the periphery of the tumor having "Cannonball"-like configuration can also be encountered[1] (Fig. 1A, B). These tumors are usually negative for myoepithelial markers.[4] However, p63 stains the squamous component with nonmyoepithelial-like diffuse staining pattern. Therefore, other myoepithelial markers are required to confirm the invasive nature of the tumor (Fig. 1C–E). The radiologic imaging (mammography or ultrasound) of LGASC is nonspecific with the mammography usually demonstrating ill-defined infiltrating lesion (Fig. 1F).

Fibromatosis-Like Metaplastic Carcinoma
The FLMC, as the name implies, has similar histologic morphology to breast fibromatosis. FLMC may show epithelioid or squamous cell differentiation and may have ductal carcinoma in situ (DCIS). When these histologic features are absent, IHC staining with epithelial markers (cytokeratin [CK] and p63) can be helpful to differentiate between these 2 lesions (Fig. 2).[5,6] The tumor cells are spindle and bland with rare, if any, mitotic figures, arranged in a wavy, interlacing fascicle or long fascicle with fingerlike extensions infiltrating the adjacent breast tissue. The tumor has infiltrating borders with a background of varying degrees of collagenization.[1] FLMC and SpCC are spectrum of the spindle cell neoplasm with substantial difference in the outcomes and treatment. Some cases could pose a challenge for the pathologist to classify. The degree of nuclear atypia, the mitotic count, and percentage of spindle cell component seem to help subclassify these tumors.[7–10] In the author's opinion, when in doubt, the case should be discussed in a multidisciplinary approach.

Squamous Cell Carcinoma
Primary breast SqCC could be pure, mixed with invasive carcinoma of no special type (NST) (high-grade adenosquamous carcinoma) or metaplastic carcinoma with

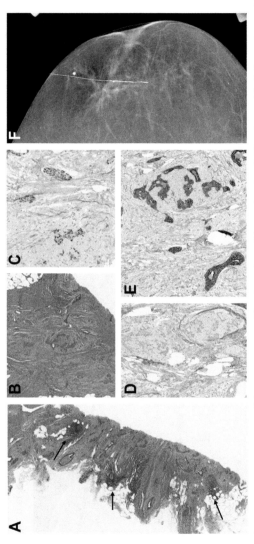

Fig. 1. Low-grade adenosquamous carcinoma. (*A*) Scanning magnification of core biopsy showing infiltrating epithelial neoplasm within a background of dense stroma; note the aggregates of lymphocytes at the periphery of the tumor (*arrows*) (H&E); (*B*) higher magnification image showing both components of infiltrating glandular and squamous clusters of cells in a background of sclerotic and desmoplastic stroma (H&E, 4x); (*C*) p63 staining showing diffuse nonmyoepithelial-like staining pattern (10x); (*D*) smooth muscle myosin image showing lack of myoepithelial cell layer in both squamous and glandular components, confirming invasion (5x); (*E*) cytokeratin 5/6 image showing diffuse staining in both the squamous and glandular components (10x); (*F*) mammography image showing ill-defined infiltrating tumor in the upper part of the breast.

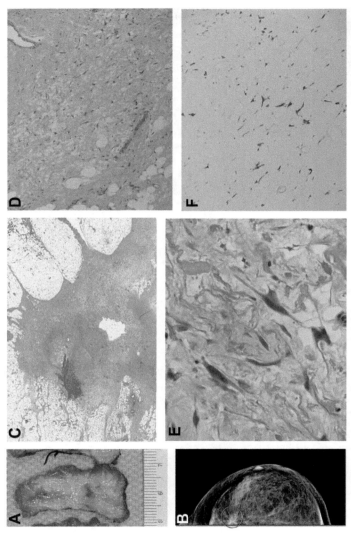

Fig. 2. Fibromatosis-like metaplastic carcinoma. (*A*) Gross image showing white fibrotic infiltrating lesion; (*B*) mammography showing irregular deeply seated lesion in the upper half of the breast; (*C*) scanning magnification of the tumor showing infiltrating fingerlike projections into the surrounding adipose tissue, corresponding to the gross image (H&E); (*D*) high power magnification showing infiltrating bland spindle cells with background of collage fibers (20x, H&E); (*E*) occasional intermediate to high atypical nuclei (60x, H&E); (*F*) pancytokeratin (AE1/3) IHC stain decorating the tumor cells (20x).

pseudoangiomatous acantholytic pattern. Moreover, SpCC could have a component of squamous differentiation. Pure SqCC usually presents as cystic mass lined up with squamous cells with varying degrees of differentiation. The periphery of the tumor shows infiltration into the surrounding stroma in forms of sheets, cords, or nests (**Fig. 3**). Some investigators classify this tumor separately from MpBC.[11] It is important to correlate with the clinical presentation, in order to rule out skin-based SqCC, or more importantly metastatic SqCC, from other organs such as lung. High-grade adenosquamous carcinoma is composed of 2 components, adenocarcinoma (ductal) and carcinoma with squamous differentiation. They are usually intermingled and difficult to appreciate the morphologic difference. Therefore, this entity is underrecognized (**Fig. 4**). The squamous component varies in proportion with a spectrum of differentiation ranging from mature keratinizing epithelium to spindle cell or with pseudoangiomatous growth pattern. Metaplastic carcinoma with pseudoangiomatous acantholytic pattern has distinctive histologic architecture with closed or interconnected irregular spaces lined with atypical malignant squamous cells (**Fig. 5**). Some investigators classify this entity under SpCC.[3] It is important to recognize this entity, as the differential diagnosis includes angiosarcoma.[12] IHC staining can be helpful, as the tumor is usually positive for one of the CK stains (high-molecular-weight or CK5) and negative for CD34.[13]

Spindle Cell Carcinoma

The SpCC or carcinosarcoma is a spectrum of spindle neoplastic disease with varying degrees of nuclear atypia, growth patterns, and differentiation. As the name implies, the tumor has spindle cell morphology with epithelioid differentiation (**Fig. 6**A). The tumor could be pure spindle cell (**Fig. 6**B) or mixed with ductal (**Fig. 6**C), or squamous differentiation/metaplasia (**Fig. 6**D). To differentiate this tumor from the less aggressive tumor FLMC, the tumor must have intermediate or highly atypical nuclei, easily identifiable or brisk mitotic figures. The other differential diagnosis is primary or metastatic sarcoma (fibrosarcoma) when the tumor has a fascicular growth pattern (see **Fig. 6**B).[14,15] Sarcoma (primary or metastatic) is treated differently from SpCC, making the distinction clinically essential. SpCC also could have variable growth pattern in which the fascicles are long, herringbone, or interwoven (see **Fig. 6**B), to short and storiform (**Fig. 6**E).[10,14,16] Presence of DCIS (**Fig. 6**F),[10] epithelioid cells (see **Fig. 6**A), and/or expression of one of the epithelial markers favors SpCC (see

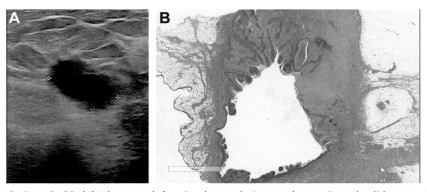

Fig. 3. Pure SqCC. (*A*) Ultrasound showing hypoechoic complex cystic and solid mass with irregular margins and some thick internal septations; (*B*) scanning magnification showing cystic formation lined up with well-differentiated SCC (H&E).

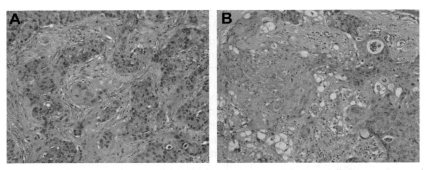

Fig. 4. Adenosquamous carcinoma. (*A*) Adenocarcinoma with intracellular mucin production intermingled with SCC (H&E, 10x); (*B*) SCC component with better differentiation (H&E, 10x).

Fig. 6E, inset). When spindle cell lesion of the breast is encountered in a CNB, MpBC diagnosis should be on the top of the differential diagnosis (see later discussion).

Metaplastic Carcinoma with Heterologous Mesenchymal Differentiation
The MCHMD, also known as heterologous metaplastic carcinoma,[3] are mixed epithelial/mesenchymal variants of metaplastic carcinoma with chondroid or osseous

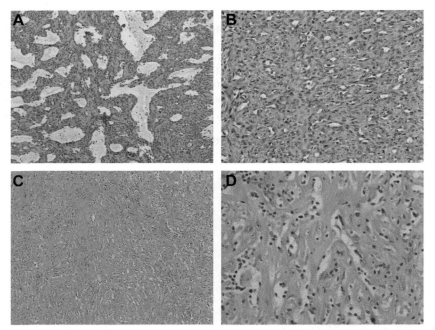

Fig. 5. SqCC acantholytic pseudoangiomatous pattern. (*A*) Dilated partially interconnected staghorn-like spaces and pseudoangiomatous growth pattern (H&E, 10x); (*B*) other areas may show only pseudoangiomatous growth pattern mimicking high-grade angiosarcoma (H&E, 20x); (*C*) another case showing collagenous background mimicking pseudoangiomatous stromal hyperplasia (H&E, 10x); (*D*) with intermediate-grade nuclear atypia (H&E, 40x).

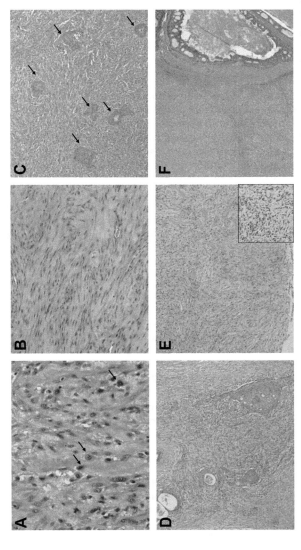

Fig. 6. SpCC. (*A*) Spindle cells with epithelioid morphology (*arrows* indicate epithelioid cells, H&E, 40x); (*B*) pure spindle cell with long sweeping fascicles (H&E, 20x); (*C*) mixed with ductal carcinoma of no special type, resembling malignant adenomyoepithelioma but lacks myoepithelial staining (*arrows* indicate ductal component, H&E, 10x); (*D*) mixed with SqCC (H&E, 10x); (*E*) pure spindle cell with short storiform fascicles (H&E, 10x; inset pancytokeratin AE1/3 staining 10x); (*F*) SpCC with DCIS (H&E, 4x).

differentiation.[17] The hallmark of these tumors is having heterologous elements, including chondroid, osseous, rhabdoid, or neurologic differentiation (**Fig. 7**A, B).[1] The other component of the tumor could be glandular, tubular, or squamous (**Fig. 7**C, D).[14,18,19] These components (heterologous elements and conventional breast carcinoma) could have either an abrupt transition or intervening zones of spindle cell metaplasia (**Fig. 7**C–E). In some cases, the tumor is completely composed of the heterologous elements with no epithelial differentiation. These tumors pose a challenge differentiating it from primary or metastatic sarcoma (osteosarcoma, chondrosarcoma, rhabdomyosarcoma). The only way of making the diagnosis is the positive staining of epithelial markers favoring carcinoma. In some instances, however, the definitive diagnosis might not be possible.

Mixed Metaplastic Breast Carcinoma

The MMC is defined as a carcinoma with a mixture of different histologic elements including various metaplastic components (SqSS, SpCC, MCHMD) or any of these elements and conventional breast carcinoma such as NST and lobular, among others (see **Fig. 4**A, B, **6**C, D, **7**D, **Fig. 8**). Because MpBCs have worse clinical outcomes than conventional breast carcinoma (see later discussion), it is recommended to report it as metaplastic carcinoma and mention the distinct conventional carcinoma components.[1] In the author's opinion, a percentage of each component should be mentioned when possible.

Some investigators classify carcinoma with multinucleated giant cells resembling osteoclasts and carcinoma with choriocarcinomatous morphology as MpBC.[3] However, these tumors are currently reclassified by the WHO under invasive breast carcinoma NST with special morphologic patterns.[1]

Unusual Clinical and Pathologic Presentation

Metaplastic Carcinoma Arising Within Complex Sclerosing Lesions

There are a few reports of complex sclerosing lesions (sclerosing papilloma and nipple adenoma) associated with metaplastic carcinoma.[20–23] In the largest series of 33 cases reported by Gobbi and colleagues, most of the cases had dominant spindle cell component with various degrees of atypia, with the majority having fibromatosis-like or low-grade morphology. Squamous metaplasia and low-grade glandular elements are common features (**Fig. 9**). DCIS and invasive mammary carcinoma could be seen but less common. Ten cases stained with IHC markers, all showing expression of at least one of the CK markers (HMW-CK, AE1/3, or CK7).[23] This entity is very important to recognize, as it can easily be overlooked when evaluating complex sclerosing lesions.

Approach to Spindle Cell Lesions of the Breast Detected in a Core Biopsy

Because MpBC is a major differential diagnosis for spindle cell lesions detected in a CNB, the author herein presents a short summary of the differential diagnosis and pitfalls and recommends histologic and IHC algorithmic approaches.

For histomorphology, first look for specific morphology such as epithelium (intimately admixed or separately coexisted) or vascular spaces. If the tumor is composed of pure spindle cells, evaluate the nuclear atypia. In this situation, clinical history of trauma or prior malignancy could be helpful. For imagining the borders of the tumor, well-defined versus infiltrative could narrow down the diagnosis (**Fig. 10**).

The IHC staining should be used in the context of the clinical and histologic findings; otherwise, they could be misleading. Identifying the cell lineage is the key in the IHC approach (epithelial, vascular vs other). First and foremost, MpBC should be at the

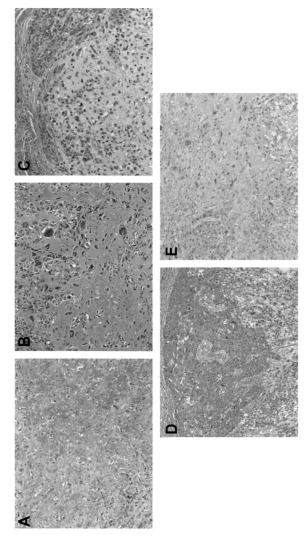

Fig. 7. MCHMD. (*A*) Matrix producing (chondroid) (H&E, 20x); (*B*) matrix producing (osteoid) (H&E, 20x); (*C*) carcinomatous (no special type) area at the periphery, note abrupt transition (H&E, 20x); (*D*) carcinomatous (squamous) area at the periphery, note abrupt transition (H&E, 20x); (*E*) zones of spindle cell metaplasia intervening between the carcinomatous and chondroid component (H&E, 20x).

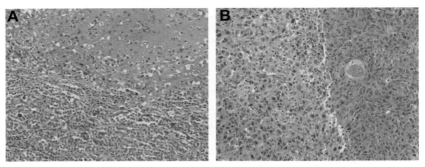

Fig. 8. Mixed metaplastic carcinoma. (*A*) MCHMD-chondroid (upper half) and lobular carcinoma (lower half) (H&E, 20x); (*B*) mixed MCHMD-chondroid (left) and SqCC (right), note the squamous pearl (H&E, 20x).

top of the differential diagnosis, and the stains should aim to rule it in or out. The most commonly used epithelial stains are AE1/3, MNF-116, HMW-CK, CK5/6, and p63.[10,24] Diffuse and strong staining patterns are usually encountered in MpBC (**Fig. 11**).

Pitfalls

- Atypical cells may be seen in benign entities such as nodular fasciitis and biopsy site, whereas some malignant entities could have bland cells such as FLMC.[1]

- It has been reported and it is in the author's experience that focal staining for keratin and p63 markers could occur in MpBC and non-MpBC tumors such as sarcoma and phyllodes tumor (PT).[25,26]

- β-catenin in PT and MpBC: Lacroix-Triki reported that all fibromatosis cases, 23% of MpBC, and 57% of PT (benign and malignant) expressed nuclear beta-catenin. However, β-catenin is usually focal when stains MpBC.[27] The author came across a case of a woman whose breast CNB had MpBC but mistakenly diagnosed as fibromatosis based on the expression of β-catenin and misinterpretation of CK stain. She presented 6 months later with double the size of the tumor. Therefore, β-catenin should be interpreted with caution in the context of the rest of the clinical and histologic findings.

MOLECULAR ALTERATIONS AND TARGET THERAPY

MpBC is usually triple-negative (estrogen receptor [ER] negative/progesterone receptor [PR] negative/HER-2/neu negative).[1,28–31] Intrinsic gene profiling classified these tumors under basal-like or claudin-low.[32,33] Further subclassification of these tumors grouped them under mesenchymal-like molecular subtype of triple-negative breast cancer (TNBC) as proposed by Lehmann and colleagues.[34] There have been many studies performed to elucidate the molecular alterations of these tumors in order to identify actionable genetic changes for potential targeted therapeutic intervention. The gene mutations are detailed in a review by González-Martínez and colleagues.[35] They reviewed 14 series with a total of 539 molecularly characterized tumors.[36–49] *TP53* was the most common mutation, followed by *PIK3CA*. *MYC* was the most amplified gene followed by *EGFR*. The most common gene loss was *CDKN2A/CDKN2B* locus (**Table 1**). There are limited data on MpBC in proper with regard to the effect of the target therapy on the actionable genes. Often, they are combined with TNBC clinical trials. However, in breast cancer in general, these monoclonal antibodies could be classified into tiers I to V and X based on the strength of the clinical evidence as

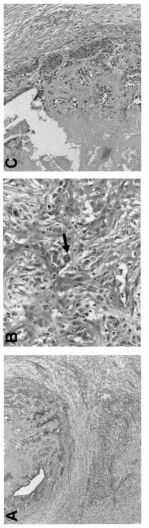

Fig. 9. Metaplastic carcinoma arising within complex sclerosing lesion. (A) Sclerosing lesion with infiltrative epithelioid cells (H&E, 4x); (B) plump fusiform and polygonal atypical tumor cells with rounded nuclei and prominent nucleoli (*arrow* indicates atypical mitotic figure) (H&E 40x); (C) squamous metaplasia at the periphery of the papilloma (H&E, 10x).

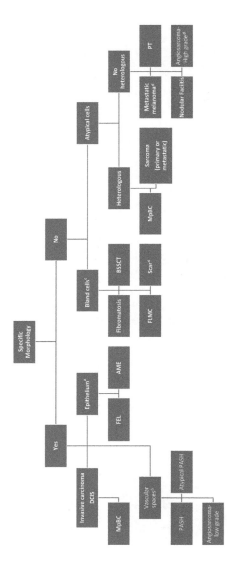

Fig. 10. Suggested algorithm of spindle cell lesion detected in core needle biopsy. [a]FEL and AME: both epithelium and stromal growths separately coexist with different proportions (AME: the spindle cells are predominantly myoepithelial). [b]IHC: CD31 positive in angiosarcoma and negative in PASH. [c]BSSCT: well-defined borders by imaging, whereas fibromatosis, FLMB, and scar: ill-defined infiltrative. [d]Scar: history of recent trauma; metastatic melanoma and metastatic sarcoma: history of the diseases; angiosarcoma: history of radiation therapy. AME, adenomamyoepithelioma; BSSCT, benign stromal spindle cell tumor (includes myofibroblastoma, spindle cell lipoma, solitary fibrous tumor); FEL, fibroepithelial lesion; FLMC, fibromatosis-like metaplastic carcinoma; MpBC, metaplastic breast carcinoma; PASH, pseudoangiomatous stromal hyperplasia; PT, phyllodes tumor.

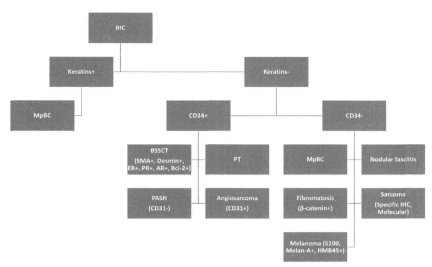

Fig. 11. Suggested IHC algorithm of spindle cell lesions detected in core needle biopsy. Keratin stains and CD34 are the major markers that can narrow down the diagnosis. Additional stains such as CD31 could be helpful. The rest of IHC should be used based on the histologic and clinical suspicion (eg, β-catenin for fibromatosis, melanoma markers, and so forth). BSSCT, benign stromal spindle cell tumor; IHC, immunohistochemistry; MpBC, metaplastic breast carcinoma; PASH, pseudoangiomatous stromal hyperplasia; PT, phyllodes tumor.

explained by Condorelli and colleagues.[50] Sporadic case reports and small clinical trials have been published illustrating variety of therapeutic approaches. The author and his colleagues reported a case of a metastatic MpBC with osseous differentiation and *BRCA1* mutation who had a marked response to liposomal doxorubicin.[51] A phase I trial on 59 patients with metastatic MpBC treated with liposomal doxorubicin, bevacizumab, with either temsirolimus or everolimus, revealed an objective response rate of 21%. All 4 patients who achieved a complete response had a mutation in the *PI3K* pathway.[52] Another observation is that MpBC patients should be tested for *BRCA* germline mutations. In addition to the benefit from adding platinum agents, they are more susceptible to Poly (ADP-ribose) polymerase inhibitors.[53]

This diverse molecular profile reflects, in part, the diversity of the histologic subtypes of MpBC. However, when dissecting through the studies, variation could be appreciated among the MpBC subtypes (SpCC, SqCC, MCHMD). SqCC and MCHMD had more frequent *TP53* mutation, whereas *PIK3CA* alterations were more frequent in SpCC.[36,46] *TERT* alteration was seen in SpCC and SqCC but not in MCHMD.[42] When MpBC was compared with non-MpBC-TNBC, the former had more *PIK3CA* alteration and less *TP53* alteration. It is worth noting that these studies focused on high-grade tumors excluding FLMC and LGASC.

TUMOR MICROENVIRONMENT AND IMMUNOTHERAPY

With the advancement of immunotherapy, few studies investigated the immune microenvironment of MpBC. Two monoclonal antibodies have been approved by the Food and Drug Administration to treat locally advanced and metastatic TNBC expressing PD-L1 with TECENTRIQ (atezolizumab) or KEYTRUDA (pembrolizumab). The corresponding IHC assays are clone SP142 and 22C3, respectively.[54,55]

Table 1
Molecular alteration in metaplastic carcinoma

Mutation	
Gene	Frequency (%)
TP53	58.7 (26–70)[a]
PIK3CA	32.8 (12–48)[a]
TERT	25
PI3K/AKT Pathway	
PTEN	12.7
PIK3R1	11.2
NF1	9.8
HRAS	8.5
AKT1	—
WNT Pathway	
APC	5
FAT1	11
DNA Repair	
BRCA1	3–15
BRCA2	2–6
ATM	2–12
Chromatin Remodeling	
KMT2D	17
ARID1A	6
Copy Number Variation (CNV)	
Amplification	
MYC	17.3
EGFR	17.2
CCND1	8.4
CCNE1	5.9
CDK4	4
CCND3	15
CCND2	5
FGFR1	5
ERBB2	4.8
RAS	5
NF1	5
PIK3CA	5
SOX2	5
AKT3	5
Gene Loss	
CDKN2A/CDKN2B	19
PTEN	14.9
RB1	6.5

[a] Median (range).

Adapted from González-Martínez S, Pérez-Mies B, Carretero-Barrio I, et al. Molecular Features of Metaplastic Breast Carcinoma: An Infrequent Subtype of Triple Negative Breast Carcinoma. Cancers (Basel). 2020;12(7):1832. Published 2020 Jul 8. https://doi.org/10.3390/cancers12071832

Tumor infiltrating lymphocytes (TILs) and PD-L1 have been extensively studied in TNBC. However, only a few focused on MpBC. Lien and colleagues scored TILs in 82 MpBC and found that 34.1% had intermediate (>10% to 60%) or high TILs (>60%) (SqCC [50%], MMC [34.1%], SpCC [30.8%], and MCHMD [14.3%]). Multivariate analysis showed that high/intermediate TILs correlated with better survival.[56] Chao and colleagues also found high TILs density in SqCC compared with other subtypes. Interestingly, in mixed MpBC/NST, TILs were denser in MpBC component than in INST component. Overall, TILs, high CD4, and high CD8 had borderline significance in correlating with clinical outcomes. In SqCC, TILs had stronger correlation with outcomes.[57]

Lien and colleagues investigated the expression of PD-L1 (SP142) in MpBC and found that it is expressed in 72% of 82 cases. When different metaplastic components were compared, the rate of expression was highest in SqCC (61.1%) and MMC (52.9%) and lowest in the chondroid component (14.3% in both the MCHMD and MMC). PD-L1 positivity did not correlate with the outcomes.[56] Other studies included MpBC as part of TNBC or breast carcinomas of all types.[44,58]

It would be clinically relevant to investigate the role of TILs in the response to neoadjuvant chemotherapy, particularly with the recent call of deescalating the therapy in patients with TNBC.

TREATMENT
Adjuvant Therapy

Classic therapeutic approaches including adjuvant chemotherapy, surgery, and radiation therapy have been previously discussed, and it is beyond the scope of this review.[59,60]

It is worth noting here in this brief review of the adjuvant treatment that as the variation in the subtypes in terms of the histopathology and the prognosis, the treatment also varies. Although high-risk MpBC is treated with surgical removal and chemotherapy, low-risk tumors (eg, LGASC and FLMC) are treated with surgical removal alone unless presented with positive lymph node.[61] Tumors that have intermediate morphology between SpCC and FLMC must be managed in a multidisciplinary approach as mentioned earlier.

Neoadjuvant Therapy

There is also a dearth of studies examining the role of neoadjuvant chemotherapy in MpBC. It is long thought that MpBC do not respond well due to the epithelial mesenchymal transformation that is commonly seen in these tumors.[62,63] Three studies with 1, 12, and 21 cases, respectively, reported low rate of pathology complete response (pCR).[64–66] In the author's experience 2 of 6 patients achieved pCR. However, in a recent study by Han and colleagues who studied 29 patients, 5 (17%) achieved pCR, most of whom were MCHMD type.[67] Overall, the rate of response is lower than the nonmetaplastic TNBC.[68] However, all these studies are retrospective and have small number of cases, making it difficult to draw any conclusions.

PROGNOSIS

There are many limitations to the published studies that investigated the clinical behavior of MpBC. MpBC is heterogeneous in terms of its clinical behavior. More specifically, these tumors can be grouped into 2 categories: low risk that includes LGASC and high risk that includes SqCC, SpCC, and MCHMD. FLMC is a unique entity, as it has intermediate risk and is considered as part of the SpCC spectrum (see later

Table 2
Studies comparing the clinical outcome between metaplastic breast carcinoma and nonmetaplastic breast carcinoma (mostly triple-negative breast cancer)

Ref	Cases (No.)	Institution	Histologic Subtypes (%)	Matching Criteria / No. Case-to-Case	DFS	OS	Multivariate Analysis	DFS (HR)	OS (HR)
Lester et al,[8] 2012	47	Single	SpCC (100)	• Age, stage, therapy (CT, RT) • One-to-one	MpBC > TNBC	Not calculated	Not calculated	Not available	Not available
Downs-Kelly et al,[18] 2009	32	Single	MCHMD (100)	• Age, stage, grade • One-to-two	MpBC > BC[a]	Not calculated	Not calculated	Not available	Not available
Jung et al,[77] 2010	35	Single	SqCC (60) MCHMD (11.4) SpCC (11.4) Mixed (14.3) LGASC (2.9)	• Grade • One-to-one	MpBC > TNBC	MpBC > TNBC	Yes	3.99	3.14
Luini et al,[78] 2007	37	Single	MCHMD (51.4) SpCC (8.1) Carcinosarcoma (24.3) SqCC (18.9) With osteoclastic giant cell (2.7)	• Grade, year of surgery, T-stage, N-stage • One-to-two	Not significant	MpBC > TNBC HR = 5.0	Not calculated	Not calculated	Not calculated
Lee et al,[79] 2012	67	Single	SqCC (52.2) SpCC (13.4) MCHMD (23.9) Mixed (7.5)[b]	• Stage • All cases	MpBC > TNBC	MpBC > TNBC	Yes	2.53	2.56
El Zein et al,[69] 2017	46	Single	MCHMD (37) SqCC (26.1) SpCC (30.4) Mixed (6.5)	• Age, stage, Nottingham grade, therapy (CT, RT) • One-to-one	MpBC > TNBC	MpBC > TNBC	Yes	1.99	Not significant
Beatty et al,[48] 2006	24	Single	SqCC (50) MCHMD (12.5)	• Date of diagnosis, age, tumor size,	Not significant	Not significant	No	Not calculated	Not calculated

Study	No.	Source	Histologic subtypes (%)	Variables	Matching	DFS[a]	OS	MpBC worse	DFS (HR)	OS (HR)
			SpCC (25), Not stated (16.5)c	node status, ER, PR, and HER2 (all cases TNBC)	Three-to-one		Not recorded	No	Not calculated	Not calculated
Rakha et al,[81] 2015	405	Multiinstitutional	SpCC (31.9)d, SqCC (21.1), Mixed SpCC/SqCC (13.5), MCHMD (28.6), FLMC (4.9)	Age, Nottingham grade, N-stage, ER and HER2; 405–285		Not significant[e]	Not recorded	No	Not calculated	Not calculated
Li et al,[70] 2019	586	SEER	Not recorded	Age, race, grade, AJCC stage, therapy (CT, RT)	One-to-three	MpBC > TNBC	MpBC > TNBC	Yes	1.42	1.36
Polamraju et al,[71] 2020	5142	NCDB (2004–2013)	Not recorded	Age, race, insurance status, T-stage, N-stage, grade, Charlson Deyo Score, year of diagnosis, income, therapy (CT, HT, RT)	All cases	Not performed	MpBC > TNBC	Yes	Not calculated	1.48
Tadros et al,[80] 2021	132	Single	SpCC (19.7), SqCC (19.7), Mixed SpCC/SqCC (22.7), MCHMD (34.1)	Age, year of surgery, type of surgery, T-stage, N-stage,	All cases	MpBC > TNBC	MpBC > TNBC	Yes	2.3	1.9

Abbreviations: DFS, disease-free survival; MpBC, metaplastic breast carcinoma; NCDB, National Cancer Data Base; OS, overall survival; SEER, Surveillance Epidemiology End Result; TNBC, triple-negative breast carcinoma.
a DFS (regional and distant).
b Two cases were not subtyped (see Table 2, Lee et al[79]).
c Cases do not add up to 100% (Beatty et al[48]).
d Only 364 cases had reported subtypes.
e Breast cancer–specific survival was calculated.

discussion). All published studies are retrospective. In the author's experience, defining MpBC is not always straightforward. For instance, in the author's published study, 28 of 81 (34.6%) reported MpBC were reclassified on review to carcinoma of NST.[69] Therefore, there is doubt about the studies that included large number of cases without pathologic review and verification.[66,70–72] On the other hand, studies with small number of cases lack statistical powers.

LGASC is largely indolent but locally aggressive. Rarely, the tumor develops lymph node or distant metastasis. In the largest series of 32 cases, the clinical outcome correlated with the tumor size.[73] FLMC is locally aggressive tumor and has the potential of distant metastasis. The risk of local recurrence could reach up to 44%.[74] Few studies reported the tumor could have potential to metastasize to other organ such as the lung,[10,75,76] although this tumor seems less aggressive than the SpCC. However, the histologic distinction between the 2 entities could be challenging. More studies are required to better define this entity, in order to better manage the patient and minimize the incidence of local or distant recurrence.

Overall, MpBC is an aggressive disease that presents as advanced disease more often than the other types of breast carcinomas. About 20% present with positive lymph node and about 25% with stage III or IV.[66,72] Often SqCC, SpCC, and MCHMD are combined in one category and compared with other tumors such as nonmetaplastic TNBC,[69–71,77–80] or NST, although matched for ER and HER2.[48,81] There are sporadic studies that investigated a single diagnosis such as SpCC[8] or MCHMD.[18] Other studies investigated if these 3 subtypes differ in the outcomes.[69,80,81] Most of these studies revealed that MpBC has worse clinical outcomes than TNBC, including 2 studies with large number of cases; the hazard ratio ranged from 1.36 and 3.99.[8,69–71,77–79] Only a single study with relatively large number of cases revealed no statistical significance between MpBC versus matching NST when only stages 1 and 2 cases were included in the analysis[81] (**Table 2**). Some studies attempted to compare the clinical outcomes between the different MpBC subtypes but limited by the small sample size.[69,82] However, Tadros and colleagues found that MCHMD had the best outcome and SqCC had the worst.[80] Rakha and colleagues revealed that SpCC, pure or mixed with SqCC, had worse clinical outcomes than SqCC or MCHMD.[81] Downs-Kelly and colleagues found that less matrix (<40%) in MCHMD signified worse clinical outcome.[18]

Comments

MpBCs are diverse group of tumors with 2 extremes, the very low risk and the very high risk. Therefore, the author recommends revising the WHO classification by proceeding the diagnoses of the least malignant tumors LGASC and FLMC with the term "low risk" and the most malignant tumors SqCC, SpCC, and MCHMD with "high risk." The high-risk tumors have the worst clinical outcomes, with some suggesting that MCHMD has better outcomes. The novel discoveries of tumor microenvironment and molecular alterations have led to the advancement in immunotherapies and target therapy. However, with few successful and promising therapies presented in the literature in the form of case reports and small clinical trials, unfortunately most of the patients succumb to this disease. Therefore, further discoveries are urgently needed.

CLINICS CARE POINTS

- High-risk MpBC has worse clinical outcomes than TNBC.
- Combining various histologic subtypes under one entity designated as MpBC is misleading.

- Some of the subtypes have the worst clinical outcomes among all breast carcinomas, whereas the other group has indolent clinical behavior.
- SpCC associated with complex sclerosing lesions could be challenging to diagnose, and the pathologists should be aware of this entity.
- Proper histomorphology interpretation and wise choices of immunohistochemistry staining could assist in rendering the correct diagnosis of spindle cell lesion of the breast.
- Target therapy and immunotherapy are promising ways to combat high-risk MpBC of various molecular alterations and up-to-date target therapy and immunotherapy.

DISCLOSURE

Breast Pathology Faculty Advisor for AstraZeneca on HER2 assay.

REFERENCES

1. Reis-Filho JS GH, McCart Reed AE, Rakha EA, et al. Metaplastic carcinoma. WHO classification of tumours of the breast. 5th edition. Lyon (France): International Agency for Research on Cancer (IARC); 2019. p. 134–8.
2. Rosen PP, Ernsberger D. Low-grade adenosquamous carcinoma. A variant of metaplastic mammary carcinoma. Am J Surg Pathol 1987;11(5):351–8.
3. Brogi E. Carcinoma with Metaplasia. In: Rosen PP, editor. Rosen's breast pathology. 5th edition. Mexico: Wolters Kluwer; 2021. p. 592–649.
4. Kawaguchi K, Shin SJ. Immunohistochemical staining characteristics of low-grade adenosquamous carcinoma of the breast. Am J Surg Pathol 2012;36(7):1009–20.
5. Dwyer JB, Clark BZ. Low-grade fibromatosis-like spindle cell carcinoma of the breast. Arch Pathol Lab Med 2015;139(4):552–7.
6. Rungta S, Kleer CG. Metaplastic carcinomas of the breast: diagnostic challenges and new translational insights. Arch Pathol Lab Med 2012;136(8):896–900.
7. Davis WG, Hennessy B, Babiera G, et al. Metaplastic sarcomatoid carcinoma of the breast with absent or minimal overt invasive carcinomatous component: a misnomer. Am J Surg Pathol 2005;29(11):1456–63.
8. Lester TR, Hunt KK, Nayeemuddin KM, et al. Metaplastic sarcomatoid carcinoma of the breast appears more aggressive than other triple receptor-negative breast cancers. Breast Cancer Res Treat 2012;131(1):41–8.
9. Zhu H, Li K, Dong DD, et al. Spindle cell metaplastic carcinoma of breast: A clinicopathological and immunohistochemical analysis. Asia-Pacific J Clin Oncol 2017;13(2):e72–8.
10. Carter MR, Hornick JL, Lester S, et al. Spindle cell (sarcomatoid) carcinoma of the breast: a clinicopathologic and immunohistochemical analysis of 29 cases. Am J Surg Pathol 2006;30(3):300–9.
11. Hoda SA. Squamous Cell Carcinoma. In: Rosen PP, editor. Rosen's breast pathology. 5th edition. Mexico: Wolters Kluwer; 2021. p. 650–64.
12. Eusebi V, Lamovec J, Cattani MG, et al. Acantholytic variant of squamous-cell carcinoma of the breast. Am J Surg Pathol 1986;10(12):855–61.
13. Aulmann S, Schnabel PA, Helmchen B, et al. Immunohistochemical and cytogenetic characterization of acantholytic squamous cell carcinoma of the breast. Virchows Arch 2005;446(3):305–9.
14. Wargotz ES, Deos PH, Norris HJ. Metaplastic carcinomas of the breast. II. Spindle cell carcinoma. Hum Pathol 1989;20(8):732–40.

15. Pitts WC, Rojas VA, Gaffey MJ, et al. Carcinomas with metaplasia and sarcomas of the breast. Am J Clin Pathol 1991;95(5):623–32.
16. Gersell DJ, Katzenstein AL. Spindle cell carcinoma of the breast. A clinocopathologic and ultrastructural study. Hum Pathol 1981;12(6):550–61.
17. Fattaneh AT. Uncommon Variants of Carcinoma. In: AFIP, editor. AFIP atlas of tumor pathology-tumors of the mammary gland, vol. 10, 4th edition. Washington, DC: Sliver Spring; 2009. p. 217–40.
18. Downs-Kelly E, Nayeemuddin KM, Albarracin C, et al. Matrix-producing carcinoma of the breast: an aggressive subtype of metaplastic carcinoma. Am J Surg Pathol 2009;33(4):534–41.
19. Oberman HA. Metaplastic carcinoma of the breast. A clinicopathologic study of 29 patients. Am J Surg Pathol 1987;11(12):918–29.
20. Pastolero GC, Bowler L, Meads GE. Intraductal papilloma associated with metaplastic carcinoma of the breast. Histopathology 1997;31(5):488–90.
21. Pitt MA, Wells S, Eyden BP. Carcinosarcoma arising in a duct papilloma. Histopathology 1995;26(1):81–4.
22. Denley H, Pinder SE, Tan PH, et al. Metaplastic carcinoma of the breast arising within complex sclerosing lesion: a report of five cases. Histopathology 2000; 36(3):203–9.
23. Gobbi H, Simpson JF, Jensen RA, et al. Metaplastic spindle cell breast tumors arising within papillomas, complex sclerosing lesions, and nipple adenomas. Mod Pathol 2003;16(9):893–901.
24. Lee AH. Recent developments in the histological diagnosis of spindle cell carcinoma, fibromatosis and phyllodes tumour of the breast. Histopathology 2008; 52(1):45–57.
25. Cimino-Mathews A, Sharma R, Illei PB, et al. A subset of malignant phyllodes tumors express p63 and p40: a diagnostic pitfall in breast core needle biopsies. Am J Surg Pathol 2014;38(12):1689–96.
26. Chia Y, Thike AA, Cheok PY, et al. Stromal keratin expression in phyllodes tumours of the breast: a comparison with other spindle cell breast lesions. J Clin Pathol 2012;65(4):339–47.
27. Lacroix-Triki M, Geyer FC, Lambros MB, et al. β-catenin/Wnt signalling pathway in fibromatosis, metaplastic carcinomas and phyllodes tumours of the breast. Mod Pathol 2010;23(11):1438–48.
28. Abouharb S, Moulder S. Metaplastic breast cancer: clinical overview and molecular aberrations for potential targeted therapy. Curr Oncol Rep 2015;17(3):431.
29. Reis-Filho JS, Milanezi F, Steele D, et al. Metaplastic breast carcinomas are basal-like tumours. Histopathology 2006;49(1):10–21.
30. Schroeder MC, Rastogi P, Geyer CE Jr, et al. Early and Locally Advanced Metaplastic Breast Cancer: Presentation and Survival by Receptor Status in Surveillance, Epidemiology, and End Results (SEER) 2010-2014. Oncologist 2018; 23(4):481–8.
31. Rakha EA, Coimbra ND, Hodi Z, et al. Immunoprofile of metaplastic carcinomas of the breast. Histopathology 2017;70(6):975–85.
32. Prat A, Parker JS, Karginova O, et al. Phenotypic and molecular characterization of the claudin-low intrinsic subtype of breast cancer. Breast Cancer Res 2010; 12(5):R68.
33. Weigelt B, Kreike B, Reis-Filho JS. Metaplastic breast carcinomas are basal-like breast cancers: a genomic profiling analysis. Breast Cancer Res Treat 2009; 117(2):273–80.

34. Lehmann BD, Bauer JA, Chen X, et al. Identification of human triple-negative breast cancer subtypes and preclinical models for selection of targeted therapies. J Clin Invest 2011;121(7):2750–67.
35. González-Martínez S, Pérez-Mies B, Carretero-Barrio I, et al. Molecular features of metaplastic breast carcinoma: an infrequent subtype of triple negative breast carcinoma. Cancers 2020;12(7):1832.
36. Piscuoglio S, Ng CKY, Geyer FC, et al. Genomic and transcriptomic heterogeneity in metaplastic carcinomas of the breast. NPJ breast cancer 2017;3:48.
37. Vranic S, Stafford P, Palazzo J, et al. Molecular Profiling of the Metaplastic Spindle Cell Carcinoma of the Breast Reveals Potentially Targetable Biomarkers. Clin Breast Cancer 2020;20(4):326–31.e1.
38. McCart Reed AE, Kalaw E, Nones K, et al. Phenotypic and molecular dissection of metaplastic breast cancer and the prognostic implications. J Pathol 2019; 247(2):214–27.
39. Zhai J, Giannini G, Ewalt MD, et al. Molecular characterization of metaplastic breast carcinoma via next-generation sequencing. Hum Pathol 2019;86:85–92.
40. Tray N, Taff J, Singh B, et al. Metaplastic breast cancers: Genomic profiling, mutational burden and tumor-infiltrating lymphocytes. Breast 2019;44:29–32.
41. Afkhami M, Schmolze D, Yost SE, et al. Mutation and immune profiling of metaplastic breast cancer: Correlation with survival. PLoS One 2019;14(11):e0224726.
42. Krings G, Chen YY. Genomic profiling of metaplastic breast carcinomas reveals genetic heterogeneity and relationship to ductal carcinoma. Mod Pathol 2018; 31(11):1661–74.
43. Ng CKY, Piscuoglio S, Geyer FC, et al. The Landscape of Somatic Genetic Alterations in Metaplastic Breast Carcinomas. Clin Cancer Res 2017;23(14):3859–70.
44. Joneja U, Vranic S, Swensen J, et al. Comprehensive profiling of metaplastic breast carcinomas reveals frequent overexpression of programmed death-ligand 1. J Clin Pathol 2017;70(3):255–9.
45. Edenfield J, Schammel C, Collins J, et al. Metaplastic breast cancer: molecular typing and identification of potential targeted therapies at a single institution. Clin Breast Cancer 2017;17(1):e1–10.
46. Ross JS, Badve S, Wang K, et al. Genomic profiling of advanced-stage, metaplastic breast carcinoma by next-generation sequencing reveals frequent, targetable genomic abnormalities and potential new treatment options. Arch Pathol Lab Med 2015;139(5):642–9.
47. Hayes MJ, Thomas D, Emmons A, et al. Genetic changes of Wnt pathway genes are common events in metaplastic carcinomas of the breast. Clin Cancer Res 2008;14(13):4038–44.
48. Beatty JD, Atwood M, Tickman R, et al. Metaplastic breast cancer: clinical significance. Am J Surg 2006;191(5):657–64.
49. Reis-Filho JS, Pinheiro C, Lambros MB, et al. EGFR amplification and lack of activating mutations in metaplastic breast carcinomas. J Pathol 2006;209(4):445–53.
50. Condorelli R, Mosele F, Verret B, et al. Genomic alterations in breast cancer: level of evidence for actionability according to ESMO Scale for Clinical Actionability of molecular Targets (ESCAT). Ann Oncol 2019;30(3):365–73.
51. Hamad L, Khoury T, Vona K, et al. A case of metaplastic breast cancer with prolonged response to single agent liposomal doxorubicin. Cureus 2016;8(1):e454.
52. Basho RK, Yam C, Gilcrease M, et al. Comparative effectiveness of an mtor-based systemic therapy regimen in advanced, metaplastic and nonmetaplastic triple-negative breast cancer. Oncologist 2018;23(11):1300–9.

53. Robson M, Im SA, Senkus E, et al. Olaparib for metastatic breast cancer in patients with a germline BRCA mutation. N Engl J Med 2017;377(6):523–33.
54. Schmid P, Adams S, Rugo HS, et al. Atezolizumab and Nab-paclitaxel in advanced triple-negative breast cancer. N Engl J Med 2018;379(22):2108–21.
55. Cortes J, Cescon DW, Rugo HS, et al. KEYNOTE-355: Randomized, double-blind, phase III study of pembrolizumab + chemotherapy versus placebo + chemotherapy for previously untreated locally recurrent inoperable or metastatic triple-negative breast cancer. J Clin Oncol 2020;38(15_suppl):1000.
56. Lien HC, Lee YH, Chen IC, et al. Tumor-infiltrating lymphocyte abundance and programmed death-ligand 1 expression in metaplastic breast carcinoma: implications for distinct immune microenvironments in different metaplastic components. Virchows Arch 2020;478(4):669–78.
57. Chao X, Liu L, Sun P, et al. Immune parameters associated with survival in metaplastic breast cancer. Breast Cancer Res 2020;22(1):92.
58. Dill EA, Gru AA, Atkins KA, et al. PD-L1 Expression and Intratumoral Heterogeneity Across Breast Cancer Subtypes and Stages: An Assessment of 245 Primary and 40 Metastatic Tumors. Am J Surg Pathol 2017;41(3):334–42.
59. Drekolias D, Mamounas EP. Metaplastic breast carcinoma: Current therapeutic approaches and novel targeted therapies. Breast J 2019;25(6):1192–7.
60. Reddy TP, Rosato RR, Li X, et al. A comprehensive overview of metaplastic breast cancer: clinical features and molecular aberrations. Breast Cancer Res 2020; 22(1):121.
61. Network NCC. Breast Cancer (Version 5.2021). Available at: https://www.nccn. org/guidelines/guidelines-detail?category=1&id=1419. Accessed May 4, 2021.
62. Kalluri R, Weinberg RA. The basics of epithelial-mesenchymal transition. J Clin Invest 2009;119(6):1420–8.
63. Sarrió D, Rodriguez-Pinilla SM, Hardisson D, et al. Epithelial-mesenchymal transition in breast cancer relates to the basal-like phenotype. Cancer Res 2008; 68(4):989–97.
64. Takuwa H, Ueno T, Ishiguro H, et al. A case of metaplastic breast cancer that showed a good response to platinum-based preoperative chemotherapy. Breast Cancer 2014;21(4):504–7.
65. Chen IC, Lin CH, Huang CS, et al. Lack of efficacy to systemic chemotherapy for treatment of metaplastic carcinoma of the breast in the modern era. Breast Cancer Res Treat 2011;130(1):345.
66. Hennessy BT, Giordano S, Broglio K, et al. Biphasic metaplastic sarcomatoid carcinoma of the breast. Ann Oncol 2006;17(4):605–13.
67. Han M, Salamat A, Zhu L, et al. Metaplastic breast carcinoma: a clinical-pathologic study of 97 cases with subset analysis of response to neoadjuvant chemotherapy. Mod Pathol 2019;32(6):807–16.
68. Huang M, O'Shaughnessy J, Zhao J, et al. Association of pathologic complete response with long-term survival outcomes in triple-negative breast cancer: a meta-analysis. Cancer Res 2020;80(24):5427–34.
69. El Zein D, Hughes M, Kumar S, et al. Metaplastic carcinoma of the breast is more aggressive than triple-negative breast cancer: a study from a single institution and review of literature. Clin Breast Cancer 2017;17(5):382–91.
70. Li Y, Zhang N, Zhang H, et al. Comparative prognostic analysis for triple-negative breast cancer with metaplastic and invasive ductal carcinoma. J Clin Pathol 2019;72(6):418–24.
71. Polamraju P, Haque W, Cao K, et al. Comparison of outcomes between metaplastic and triple-negative breast cancer patients. Breast 2020;49:8–16.

72. Pezzi CM, Patel-Parekh L, Cole K, et al. Characteristics and treatment of meta-plastic breast cancer: analysis of 892 cases from the National Cancer Data Base. Ann Surg Oncol 2007;14(1):166–73.
73. Van Hoeven KH, Drudis T, Cranor ML, et al. Low-grade adenosquamous carci-noma of the breast. A clinocopathologic study of 32 cases with ultrastructural analysis. Am J Surg Pathol 1993;17(3):248–58.
74. Gobbi H, Simpson JF, Borowsky A, et al. Metaplastic breast tumors with a domi-nant fibromatosis-like phenotype have a high risk of local recurrence. Cancer 1999;85(10):2170–82.
75. Sneige N, Yaziji H, Mandavilli SR, et al. Low-grade (fibromatosis-like) spindle cell carcinoma of the breast. Am J Surg Pathol 2001;25(8):1009–16.
76. Kurian KM, Al-Nafussi A. Sarcomatoid/metaplastic carcinoma of the breast: a clinicopathological study of 12 cases. Histopathology 2002;40(1):58–64.
77. Jung SY, Kim HY, Nam BH, et al. Worse prognosis of metaplastic breast cancer patients than other patients with triple-negative breast cancer. Breast Cancer Res Treat 2010;120(3):627–37.
78. Luini A, Aguilar M, Gatti G, et al. Metaplastic carcinoma of the breast, an unusual disease with worse prognosis: the experience of the European Institute of Oncology and review of the literature. Breast Cancer Res Treat 2007;101(3): 349–53.
79. Lee H, Jung SY, Ro JY, et al. Metaplastic breast cancer: clinicopathological fea-tures and its prognosis. J Clin Pathol 2012;65(5):441–6.
80. Tadros AB, Sevilimedu V, Giri DD, et al. Survival outcomes for metaplastic breast cancer differ by histologic subtype. Ann Surg Oncol 2021;28(8):4245–53.
81. Rakha EA, Tan PH, Varga Z, et al. Prognostic factors in metaplastic carcinoma of the breast: a multi-institutional study. Br J Cancer 2015;112(2):283–9.
82. Leyrer CM, Berriochoa CA, Agrawal S, et al. Predictive factors on outcomes in metaplastic breast cancer. Breast Cancer Res Treat 2017;165(3):499–504.

Update on Ovarian Sex Cord–Stromal Tumors

Zehra Ordulu, MD

KEYWORDS

- Ovary • Sex cord-stromal tumor • Microcystic stromal tumor
- Adult granulosa cell tumor • Sertoli–Leydig cell tumor • Gynandroblastoma • FOXL2
- DICER1 • Juvenile Granulosa cell tumor

KEY POINTS

- Molecular testing might be useful in the diagnosis of morphologically challenging tumors, as illustrated by the *FOXL2* mutation testing for the differential diagnosis of adult granulosa cell tumor.
- Although adult granulosa cell tumors are typically characterized by *FOXL2* mutation, a minor subset is *FOXL2* wild type and the latter may be enriched in tumors admixed with other sex cord–stromal tumor morphologies.
- Molecular subtypes of Sertoli–Leydig cell tumors include *DICER1*-mutated, *FOXL2*-mutated, and *DICER1* and *FOXL2* wild type.
- Increasing molecular data combined with clinical and morphologic findings may result in revisiting some of the historical concepts such as gynandroblastomas, a subset of which may represent Sertoli-Leydig cell tumors with juvenile granulosa-like follicles.

INTRODUCTION

More than one-half of a century after the publication of the fundamental book "Endocrine Pathology of the Ovary" mainly focusing on ovarian sex cord–stromal tumors (SCSTs) by Drs Morris and Scully,[1] these neoplasms remain to be diagnostically challenging to the practicing pathologist due to their rarity, which is disproportionate to the variety in their morphology.[2–4] Although staining with sex cord–stromal markers (eg, WT1, SF1, FOXL2, inhibin, calretinin) and the lack of EMA expression can ascertain the lineage, immunohistochemistry is of limited value in further distinguishing among the SCST categories.[5–7] As in any other tumor type, molecular advances in this field over the last decade can provide an additional layer of information that may be beneficial for their diagnosis and clinical management.[7–9] Herein, ovarian SCSTs with

This article originally appeared in *Surgical Pathology Clinics* Volume 15 Issue 2, June 2022.
Department of Pathology, Immunology and Laboratory Medicine, University of Florida, 1345 Center Drive, Box 100275, Gainesville, FL 32610, USA
E-mail address: mordulusahin@ufl.edu

Clin Lab Med 43 (2023) 245–274
https://doi.org/10.1016/j.cll.2023.03.001
0272-2712/23/Published by Elsevier Inc.

recent clinicopathologic and genetic updates are discussed in line with their 2020 World Health Organization classification.[10]

PURE STROMAL TUMORS
Fibroma

Fibromas, the most common ovarian stromal tumors, show fascicular growth of bland spindled to ovoid cells with scant cytoplasm and varying degrees of intercellular collagen.[10,11] They typically present as a unilateral mass in patients older than 30 and may be associated with ascites and pleural effusion (Meigs' syndrome) (**Table 1**).[12] Bilateral fibromas in younger patients occur in the setting of Gorlin (nevoid

Table 1 World Health Organization classification of pure stromal tumors and corresponding clinical and molecular features				
Histologic Classification (Pure Stromal)	Presentation	Average Age (Range)[a]	Altered Gene(s)	Syndromic Association
Fibroma	Pelvic mass, ascites and pleural effusion (Meigs' syndrome)	48 (any age, typically >30)	IDH1, cellular fibroma: STK11[b] and PTCH1[b]	Gorlin (SUFU, PTCH1), Ollier (IDH1)
Thecoma	Endocrine (E > A)	49.6–59.5 (16–81)	Rarely FOXL2[b]	NA
LTSP	Bilateral pelvic masses, bowel obstruction, ascites	28 (10 mo to 85 y)	NA	NA
SST	Pelvic mass, endocrine (E > A), rarely Meigs' syndrome	26 (12–63)	GLI2 fusions (FHL2 most common partner)	Gorlin (SUFU, PTCH1)
MST	Pelvic mass	45 (23–71)	CTNNB1, APC	FAP (APC)
SRST	Pelvic mass	36 (21–83)	CTNNB1[b]	NA
LCT	Endocrine (A > E)	58 (32–82)	NA	NA
SCT	Endocrine (A > E > Cushing syndrome), pelvic mass	43 (rare before puberty, wide range)	NA	Von Hippel–Lindau syndrome (VHL)
Ovarian fibrosarcoma	Pelvic mass	Postmenopausal	NA	Gorlin (SUFU, PTCH1), Maffucci (IDH1)

Abbreviations: A, androgenic; E, estrogenic; FAP, familial adenomatous polyposis; LTSP, luteinized thecoma with sclerosing peritonitis; LCT, Leydig cell tumor; MST, microcystic stromal tumor; mo: months, NA, not available; SCT, steroid cell tumor, SRST, signet ring stromal tumor, SST, sclerosing stromal tumor, y: years.
[a] In years unless specified otherwise.
[b] Controversial, see relevant subtitle.

basal cell carcinoma) syndrome.[13] Among the individuals with Gorlin syndrome, those with germline *SUFU* alterations are more likely to have ovarian fibromas than those with *PTCH1*.[14] In addition, a single cellular fibroma case was reported to have an *IDH1* mutation in a patient with Ollier disease.[15] Common somatic alterations in fibromas include imbalances of chromosomes 4, 9, 12, and 19.[16–21] Of note, a single study showed that 50% of cellular fibromas have concurrent 9q22.3 and 19p13.3 loss of heterozygosity (LOH).[19] While 19p13.3 LOH was seen in usual fibromas and other SCSTs (albeit less frequently), 9q22.3 LOH was not detected in these tumors.[18,19] One of the conclusions from this study[19] was the potential involvement of *PTCH1* (9q22.3) and *STK11* (19p13.3) in cellular fibromas. However, these results should be interpreted with caution because the specific microsatellite markers that were lost did not encompass either *PTCH1* or *STK11*, and they were only on the same respective chromosome arms.

The morphologic diagnosis of a fibroma is usually straightforward. However, cellular fibromas, especially those that are mitotically active ($\geq$4 mitoses/10 high-power field) (MACFs), may be challenging to differentiate from their malignant counterparts (fibrosarcoma)[11,22] and adult granulosa cell tumors (AGCTs). Although fibrosarcoma (exceedingly rare) and MACF both have increased mitotic rate and cellularity, the former also has moderate to severe atypia as opposed to the bland cytology of MACFs. In addition, fibrosarcoma is typically more homogenously cellular, whereas MACF can have usual fibroma-like foci admixed with the more cellular component.[3,22] In contrast, the distinction of cellular fibroma from AGCT can be extremely difficult based on just morphology. Reticulin staining around individual cells favors the diagnosis of a fibroma in this setting (**Fig. 1**A, B). However, the interpretation of this stain might be problematic, as illustrated by a study having an indeterminate reticulin pattern in about one-third of the analyzed SCSTs.[23] A more definitive approach is to perform *FOXL2* mutation analysis for the characteristic p.C134W variant seen in up to greater than 95% of AGCTs,[24] whereas it is negative in cellular fibromas.[25] Last, it is interesting to note that one case, classified by the authors as MACF, was shown to have a novel *FOXL2* mutation (p.R144W).[23]

Diagnostic Pitfall: Cellular Fibroma versus Adult Granulosa Cell Tumors

- Reticulin around individual cells favors fibroma
- Consider *FOXL2* mutation testing if reticulin is indeterminate

---

Thecoma

Thecomas have a diffuse to nodular growth pattern, occasionally with hyaline plaques, calcification, and sclerosis, and cells with bland nuclei, pale gray cytoplasm with indistinct cytoplasmic membranes.[26,27] They present with estrogenic symptoms in peri or postmenopausal women rather than symptoms of a pelvic mass.[28] Calcified thecomas tend to occur in younger women.[29] A unique molecular alteration specific for thecomas has not been identified; however, this may have been confounded by the single gene mutation based nature of the molecular assays used in the majority of relevant literature. A small subset of thecomas is reported to have the *FOXL2* mutation typical of AGCTs, which will be discussed further elsewhere in this article.[7,24,30–32]

It is well-established that thecomas have a morphologic overlap with fibromas. In tumors exhibiting both morphologies, the classification should be done based on predominant morphology, although some may also use the term fibrothecoma.[21] In contrast, AGCT represent a more challenging and clinically significant differential

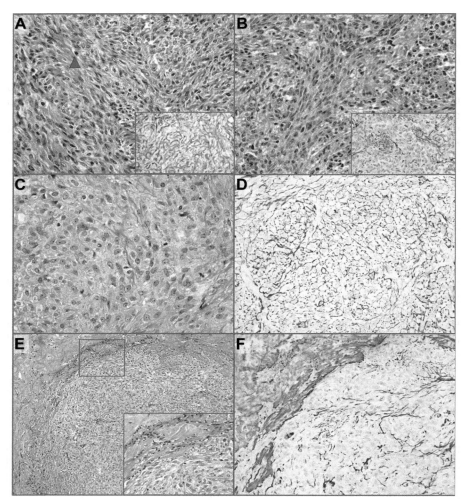

Fig. 1. (*A*) Mitotically active cellular fibroma (*arrowhead*, mitosis; *inset*, reticulin stain wrapping individual cells). (*B*) Diffuse AGCT (*inset*, reticulin stain showing nesting around tumor cell groups with loss of pericellular staining). (*C*) Thecoma with abundant pale gray cytoplasm. (*D*) Reticulin corresponding to the thecoma in (*C*), wrapping individual cells. (*E*) AGCT with thecoma-like foci (*inset*, high-power view to show the morphologic distinction between thecoma-like areas in the majority of the nodule and granulosa-like areas at the periphery of the nodule). (*F*) Reticulin corresponding to the tumor in (*E*) with nested pattern in both thecoma-like and granulosa-like areas.

diagnosis, given its malignant potential. A recent series describing AGCTs with thecoma-like foci[33] reported that these tumors were usually nodular and had cells with moderately abundant pale-gray cytoplasm. The thecomatous versus granulosa nature of these cells were almost indistinguishable without the aid of a reticulin stain (**Fig. 1C–F**). In addition, the classic granulosa morphology with spindled to ovoid cells with scant cytoplasm was usually a minority of the tumor (typically at the periphery of the nodules) (see **Fig. 1E**). Therefore, based on hematoxylin and eosin staining alone, the granulosa component might be underestimated initially and, not surprisingly, 40% of the tumors in this series had the referral diagnosis as a thecoma. Overall, the authors highlighted the importance of reticulin staining particularly in the setting of thecomatous tumors with nodular architecture. These AGCTs with thecoma-like foci are perhaps akin to the historical granulosa theca cell tumors[34,35] (further discussed under gynandroblastoma), which were shown to have the *FOXL2* mutation in 50% of the cases.[36] Taken together, the possibility of the previously mentioned rare thecomas with the *FOXL2* mutation actually representing an AGCT cannot be excluded. In fact, one of them was reported to have a minor granulosa cell component[24] and another study[31] reported an abdominal tumor with classic AGCT morphology in a woman who was diagnosed with a small ovarian thecoma 2 years prior. Both of these tumors had the same *FOXL2* mutation, suggesting that the initial thecoma was a misdiagnosed AGCT with thecoma-like foci.

Diagnostic Pitfall: Adult Granulosa Cell Tumor with Thecoma-Like Foci

- Thecoma and AGCT morphology may look indistinguishable on hematoxylin and eosin staining, causing underestimation of the granulosa component
- Reticulin staining should be used liberally for nodular thecomatous tumors (loss of pericellular reticulin staining favoring AGCT)

Sclerosing Stromal Tumor

Sclerosing stromal tumors (SSTs) have pseudolobulation, prominent ectatic vessels, and an admixture of lutein cells and fibroblasts.[37,38] They can show prominent luteinization during pregnancy[39] and rarely can be mitotically active.[38,40] They typically present with symptoms of a pelvic mass or are incidental. A single patient with Gorlin syndrome was reported to have SST.[41] Somatic alterations in SSTs include trisomy 12.[42,43] Recently, *GLI2* fusions have been detected in these tumors (most common partner: *FHL2*).[44]

Most SSTs are readily recognizable, but sometimes other SCSTs including fibromas, thecomas, luteinized thecoma with sclerosing peritonitis (**Fig 2**A), and steroid cell tumors (particularly in pregnant patients) enter in the differential diagnosis, as well as solitary fibrous tumors.[45,46] The unique combination of pseudolobulation, ectatic vessels, and the jumbled mixture of lutein cells and fibroblasts should prompt the diagnosis of SST[38] (**Fig. 2**B–D). For solitary fibrous tumors, STAT6 staining can provide additional reassurance given the rarity of these tumors at this site.

Microcystic Stromal Tumor and Signet Ring Stromal Tumor

Microcystic stromal tumors (MSTs) are rare and represent the most recently described SCST.[47] The classic morphologic features include solid cellular zones with microcysts that may coalesce into larger channels, intersected by fibrous stroma with hyaline plaques (**Fig. 3**A–C). The tumor cells have pale or gray cytoplasm, sometimes vacuolated, as well as round, uniform nuclei with occasional bizarre atypia. On the other hand, MSTs with nonconventional morphology might have diffuse solid, corded, and/or nested architecture of cells with eosinophilic cytoplasm and variable intracytoplasmic vacuoles with only minimal or no microcysts (**Fig. 3**D).[48,131] Patients usually present with symptoms of a pelvic mass, typically unilateral. Bilateral ovarian involvement has been rarely reported.[50] MSTs may be seen in the setting of familial adenomatous polyposis with germline *APC* mutations and a second hit in the MST.[51,52] The most common somatic mutations involve *CTNNB1* and, less frequently, *APC*. They lack mutations in *FOXL2* and *DICER1*.[52–56] Although these tumors are generally considered benign, 2 cases

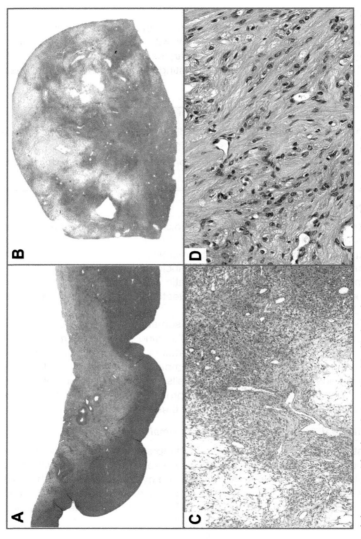

Fig. 2. (A) Luteinized thecoma with sclerosing peritonitis displays characteristic cerebriform hypercellularity at the periphery of the ovarian stroma. (B–D) SST is characterized by pseudolobulation at low power view (B), ectatic vessels and alternating hypocellular and hypercellular areas (C), and a mixture of luteinized cells and spindled cells (D).

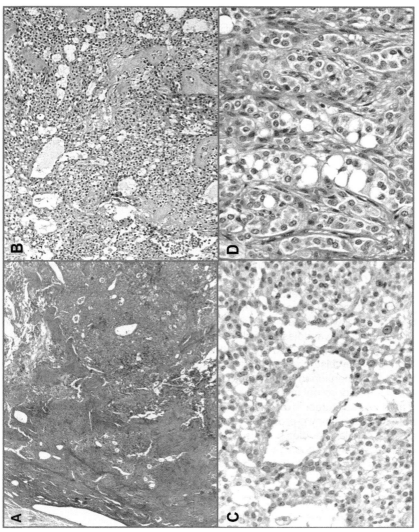

Fig. 3. Microcystic stromal tumor. (A–C) Typical morphology includes pseudolobulated architecture (A), microcysts and macrocysts with hyaline plaques in the background (B), and a monomorphic cell population with intracytoplasmic vacuoles and uniform round nuclei, forming microcysts (C). (D) Nonconventional morphology is sometimes seen, in this example featuring nests of cells with eosinophilic cytoplasm and intracytoplasmic vacuoles (Courtesy of Dr McCluggage).

with recurrence have been reported, one of which had variants of uncertain significance in *APC* and *KRAS*.[57,58] MSTs have a distinct immunohistochemical profile among the majority of SCSTs; as beta catenin and cyclin D1 stains can be used as a surrogate for the activation of the WNT signaling pathway.[54] In addition, they are positive for CD10, WT1, SF1, and FOXL2, but negative for inhibin and calretinin.[48,54]

Signet ring stromal tumors (SRSTs)[59–61] are in the differential diagnosis of nonconventional MSTs. Both of these extremely rare tumors have cellular fibromatous stroma with signet ring cells, each featuring a single clear intracellular vacuole that is negative for lipid or mucin. Interestingly, testicular SRSTs have been shown to harbor *CTNNB1* mutations and express nuclear beta catenin postulating a potential link to MST.[62] One case described as ovarian SRST and showing nuclear beta catenin has been reported.[63] Moreover, a collusion tumor consisting of SRST and steroid cell tumor also showed nuclear beta catenin expression restricted to the SRST component.[64] However, it is possible that the reported ovarian SRSTs with *CTNNB1* mutations [63,64] may actually represent nonconventional MSTs based on the provided photomicrographs. A separate study documenting bilateral SRSTs showed lack of nuclear beta catenin expression, as well as *CTNNB1* and *FOXL2* mutations,[65] a profile that is more in keeping with fibroma. Overall, it may be speculated that SRSTs represent a morphologic spectrum from fibromas with signet ring cells (*CTNNB1* wild-type) to non-conventional MSTs (*CTNNB1* mutated), and additional studies are warranted for better classification of these extremely rare tumors. With the currently available information, SRSTs usually show a signet ring cell component in a fibromatous background, whereas signet ring cells in MSTs are seen in a background of solid, nested and corded growth patterns separated by fibrous septae. MSTs do not always show the typical microcysts but when present, they help with the differential diagnosis. Of note, another rare neoplasm, solid pseudopapillary tumor of the ovary,[66,67] also has similar *CTNNB1* mutations and CD10 positivity, but should be differentiated based on morphologic features.

Another consideration for the differential of nonconventional MSTs and SRSTs is a Krukenberg tumor, which also exhibits signet ring cell morphology.[61,68–70] The mucinous nature of the vacuoles, as well as the atypia of the nuclei (which can be subtle, but often appreciable), should prompt the consideration of this possibility, which can be confirmed by histochemistry for mucicarmine and an immunostaining panel including the aforementioned markers and EMA (negative in SCSTs). Lastly, although a steroid cell tumor does not immediately come to mind as a mimicker, there is a case report of a steroid cell tumor in a patient with familial adenomatous polyposis,[71] where the photomicrographs may represent a nonconventional MST as pointed out by other authors.[52] The ancillary studies can also be used in this setting.

Molecular features and considerations for differential diagnosis of pure stromal tumors discussed herein are summarized in **BOX 1** and **BOX 2**, respectively.

Box 1
Molecular pathology features: pure stromal tumors

Fibroma
- Somatic: Chromosomal imbalances of 4, 9, 12 and 19, *IDH1* mutation
- Syndromic: Gorlin (*SUFU*, *PTCH1*), Ollier (*IDH1*) (single case report)

Thecoma
- Somatic: Small subset of cases described as harboring *FOXL2* mutation (may represent AGCT with thecoma-like foci)

Sclerosing stromal tumor
- Somatic: Trisomy 12, *GLI2* fusions (*FHL2* most common partner)
- Syndromic: Gorlin (*SUFU, PTCH1*) (single case report)

Microcystic stromal tumor
- Somatic: *CTNNB1* > *APC* mutations (mutually exclusive)
- Syndromic: Familial adenomatous polyposis (*APC*)

Box 2
Differential diagnosis: pure stromal tumors

Mitotically active cellular fibroma
- Fibrosarcomas: Moderate to severe cytologic atypia
- AGCTs: Nested reticulin, *FOXL2* mutation

Thecoma
- Fibromas: If morphologic overlap, classify based on predominant morphology
- AGCTs with thecoma-like foci: Nested reticulin, *FOXL2* mutation

Sclerosing Stromal Tumor
- Other SCSTs: The unique constellation of pseudolobulation, ectatic vessels, and the jumbled mixture of lutein cells and fibroblasts separates SSTs from mimickers that may have 1 or 2 of these findings individually and focally.
- Solitary fibrous tumor: In addition to above-mentioned morphologic criteria, STAT6 expression in solitary fibrous tumors

Microcystic stromal tumor
- The morphologic spectrum recently expanded
- Those without microcysts can mimic SRST and Krukenberg
- Positive: Beta catenin (nuclear staining), cyclin D1, CD10, WT1, FOXL2, SF1
- Negative: Inhibin, calretinin, EMA

Diagnostic Pitfall: Nonconventional Microcystic Stromal Tumor

- May be diffusely solid, nested, and corded (without obvious microcysts)
- Eosinophilic cytoplasm with occasional intracytoplasmic vacuoles
- Immunohistochemistry is helpful in confirming the diagnosis

---

PURE SEX CORD TUMORS
Adult Granulosa Cell Tumor

Accounting for 90% of malignant SCSTs of the ovary, AGCTs in their conventional form have scant cytoplasm and round to ovoid uniform nuclei with interspersed nuclear grooves. They show many architectural patterns (**Fig. 4**): diffuse, corded, trabecular, insular, and less frequently pseudopapillary, gyriform, and macrofollicular. The most distinctive morphology is microfollicular, which features with Call–Exner bodies (see **Fig. 4**A); however, this pattern is seen in a minority of cases. AGCTs typically present in perimenopausal women with abdominal pain and estrogenic symptoms (**Table 2**).[72] Although AGCTs are not recurrently associated with a syndrome, there is a single case with a germline *TP53* mutation showing multifocal intrafollicular AGCT.[73] Despite the variety in their morphology, AGCTs are molecularly homogenous tumors showing a recurrent and relatively specific *FOXL2* mutation (c.C402G; p.C134W),[24,74] which can be used for diagnostic purposes. The frequency of this

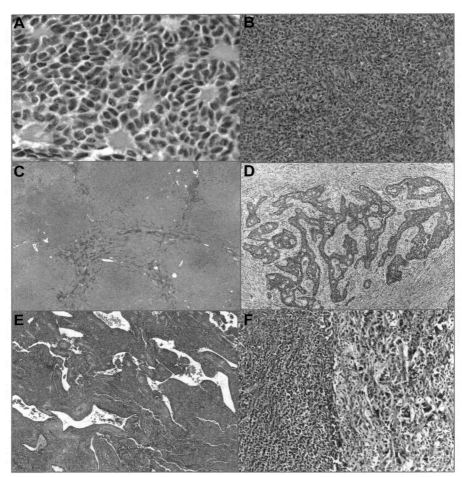

Fig. 4. Adult granulosa cell tumor shows a spectrum of morphologies. (*A*) Characteristic Call–Exner bodies (rare), (*B*) diffuse (most common), (*C*) fibrothecomatous nodules with more typical morphology at the periphery of the nodules, (*D*) trabeculated architecture in fibromatous stroma, (*E*) papillary architecture, and (*F*) high-grade transformation with a sharp demarcation between low-grade (*left*) and high-grade (*right*) components.

FOXL2 mutation in AGCTs is reported as 90% or more in most studies,[23,24,30,74–76] with only few reports showing frequencies of 60% to 80%.[77–79] These discrepancies may be attributed to technical aspects of the sequencing (quality of the DNA, tumor percentage, etc); however, it is also important to note, at least for one of these series,[78] the nature of the cohort (being predominantly consult cases) implies these tumors were morphologically more challenging than a bona fide AGCT. In fact, one of the striking findings in this study was that the *FOXL2* wild-type AGCTs were enriched for other SCST elements (further discussed under Gynandroblastoma). Of note, a recent series using whole genome sequencing found *DICER1* mutations in 2/4 *FOXL2* wild-type AGCT.[76] FOXL2 is a transcription factor regulating ovarian granulosa and follicle cell development.[80] Germline *FOXL2* loss-of-function mutations may result in premature ovarian failure in the setting of autosomal dominant blepharophimoses,

Table 2
World Health Organization classification of pure sex-cord and mixed tumors and corresponding clinical and molecular features

Histologic Classification	Presentation	Average Age (Range)[a]	Altered Gene(s)	Syndromic Association
Pure sex cord				
AGCT	Solid and cystic pelvic mass, endocrine (E > A)	50 (any age, rare in first decade)	FOXL2, KMT2D; High-grade: TP53; Recurrent: TERT	NA
JGCT	Solid and cystic pelvic mass, endocrine (prepubertal: isosexual pseudoprecocity, older: AUB)	13 (0–67)	Common: AKT1, GNAS, KMT2C, TERT rearrangement, DICER1; Rare: IDH1, FOXL2	DICER1-S, Ollier (IDH1) and Maffucci (IDH1)
Sertoli cell tumor	Pelvic mass, endocrine (E > A)	30 (any age)	Rarely DICER1	PJS (STK11)
SCTAT	Incidental, rarely progesterone	20–30 (<10–>70)	NA	PJS (STK11)
Mixed				
SLCT	Endocrine (A); Endocrine (E > A)	24.5 (15–62); 79.5 (51–90); 51 (17–74)	DICER1; FOXL2; Non-DICER1/FOXL2	DICER1-S
SCST, NOS	NA	NA	Variable based on morphology	NA
Gynandroblastoma	Abdominal pain, endocrine	24.5 (14–80)	Variable based on morphology	DICER1-S

Abbreviations: A, androgenic; AGCT, adult granulosa cell tumor; AUB, abnormal uterine bleeding; E, estrogenic; JGCT, juvenile granulosa cell tumor; NA, not available; PJS, Peutz–Jeghers syndrome; S, syndrome; SCTAT, sex cord-tumor with annular tubules; SCST, NOS, sex cord–stromal tumor, not otherwise specified; SLCT, Sertoli-Leydig cell tumor.

[a] In years.

ptosis, and epicanthus syndrome.[81] Conversely, the *FOXL2* mutation in the AGCTs is presumed to be an oncogenic activation.[82] Of note, FOXL2 immunohistochemistry should not be used as a surrogate for *FOXL2* mutation, because it is also positive in other SCSTs in the absence of *FOXL2* aberrations.[31] Therefore, this stain is useful as a biomarker of sex cord–stromal lineage, but it is not specific for AGCT.

Unlike the majority of benign stromal tumors, AGCT are of low malignant potential with approximately a 20% recurrence rate, often decades after diagnosis, thus requiring close and long-term follow-up.[83–85] Recurrent tumors are predominantly enriched in *TERT* promoter variants.[76,86–88] A clinically significant recent advance is that *FOXL2* and *TERT* promoter mutations can be detected in circulating tumor DNA, which can be used as a biomarker for disease monitoring.[89,90] Other variants implied in recurrent tumors, but not consistently documented by multiple studies, include *KMT2D* (seen in approximately 10% of AGCT), *TP53*, and *MED12* mutations, and *CDKN2A*/B homozygous deletions.[88,91,92]

Recently, a rare subset of AGCTs with high-grade transformation have been described with relatively more aggressive behavior.[93,94] The high-grade areas of the tumor have an abrupt transition from the typical low-grade morphology (see **Fig. 4F**), and are characterized by marked atypia with multinucleated cells, a high mitotic count, and often a differential p53-mutated pattern staining, which is wild type in the low-grade areas. The high-grade areas may resemble juvenile granulosa cell tumor (JGCT) with abundant eosinophilic cytoplasm and intermediate sized follicles; however, both components have the typical *FOXL2* mutation indicating a clonal AGCT origin. The authors noted that these tumors may be similar to the previously reported AGCTs with sarcomatous transformation[95–97]; however, they are different than those with occasional bizarre nuclei with no significant mitotic activity.[98,99] In addition, an earlier series[32] reported an AGCT recurrence being misdiagnosed as a high-grade serous carcinoma due to pleomorphism and p53 staining, which then was found to have the same *FOXL2* mutation with the primary AGCT tumor removed 2 years ago, thus evoking the phenomenon of high-grade transformation. Another similar report described an aggressive AGCT with rapid recurrence composed of low-grade and sarcomatoid components, the latter showing enlarged bizarre nuclei, increased mitosis, and mutated-pattern p53 expression, whereas the former with wild-type-pattern p53 staining.[97] Finally, a recent series with molecular analysis on AGCTs[76] identified a small subset (3/46) with *TP53* mutations, a high tumor mutational burden, and an increased mitotic index, recapitulating the findings of the aforementioned high-grade transformation study.[93]

Diagnostic Pitfall: Adult Granulosa Cell Tumor with High-Grade Transformation

- High-grade transformation in AGCT may mimic other pleomorphic tumors, especially if tumor is not well-sampled or is the sole morphology in a recurrence
- Patient's clinical history and careful examination of the tumor for areas with typical morphology should alleviate this caveat, and prompt further ancillary studies if necessary

---

Juvenile Granulosa Cell Tumor

JGTCs have a nodular or diffuse growth pattern with interspersed follicles of various shapes and irregular contours, usually containing basophilic secretions and set in an edematous to myxoid stroma. The cells have abundant eosinophilic cytoplasm and hyperchromatic nuclei with variable atypia (**Fig. 5**).[100] Most lesions present as a unilateral solid and cystic mass in younger patients, with an average age of 13 (wide range, most commonly in the first decade). Most of the prepubertal patients

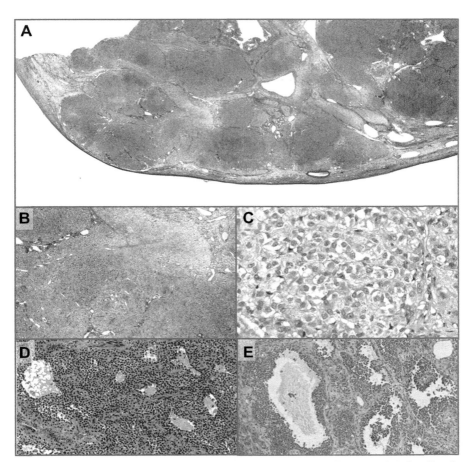

Fig. 5. (A-C) Juvenile granulosa cell tumor with multinodular architecture (A), focally sclerotic nodules (B), and (nests of cells with abundant cytoplasm and atypical nuclei (C). (D) Juvenile granulosa cell tumor follicles have variable sizes and shapes and basophilic secretions. (E) Small cell carcinoma, hypercalcemic type is an important differential diagnosis, as it can form follicle-like spaces; these are lined by small round blue neoplastic cells without polarization.

affected show isosexual pseudoprecocity, whereas older patients can have symptoms of a pelvic mass and abnormal uterine bleeding.[100] These tumors can be seen in patients with Ollier disease, Maffucci syndrome (*IDH1*),[100–102] and *DICER1* syndrome.[103] Case reports of this tumor in a patient with tuberous sclerosis[104] and another with concurrent *TP53* and *PTEN* germline mutations, have been published.[105] Activating alterations of *AKT1* (60%) and *GNAS* (30%), as well as *DICER1* (10%) mutations are recurrently identified in JGCTs,[106,107] whereas *FOXL2* mutations are rare.[24,108–110] A recent comprehensive analysis of JGCTs reported *KMT2C* and other SWI/SNF complex gene mutations, as well as *TERT* rearrangements, in addition to previously reported *AKT1* and *DICER1* mutations.[111]

The age group and the follicular growth seen in these tumors brings the differential consideration of small cell carcinoma, hypercalcemic type showing follicle-like spaces (see **Fig. 5E**) and, to a lesser extent, germ cell tumors, in particular yolk sac tumors forming cysts. However, the characteristic morphologic features and the lack of endocrine presentation in those tumors are usually enough to make a definitive diagnosis. For confirmatory purposes, EMA, and SMARCA4 can be performed to exclude small cell carcinoma, hypercalcemic type, and SALL4 for yolk sac tumors.

Molecular features and considerations for differential diagnosis of pure sex cord tumors discussed herein are summarized in **BOX 3** and **BOX 4**, respectively.

MIXED SEX CORD–STROMAL TUMORS
Sertoli–Leydig Cell Tumor

Sertoli–Leydig cell tumors (SLCTs) commonly have moderate to poorly and, less frequently, well-differentiated forms (usually seen in the pure Sertoli cell tumor setting). Differentiation depends on the presence and amount of tubular differentiation versus primitive gonadal stroma.[112] Well-differentiated forms have tubules showing no significant atypia. Moderately differentiated forms usually have a lobular pattern of Sertoli cells growing in nests (less often in tubules) with mild to moderate cytologic atypia. Leydig cells usually present at the periphery of the lobules. Poorly differentiated ones show a primitive and sarcomatoid stroma, sometimes admixed with moderately differentiated SLCT elements in the background. Retiform SLCTs have anastomosing spaces with papillary structures that are reminiscent of the rete testis. SLCTs can have heterologous elements in epithelial (carcinoid, intestinal glands) or mesenchymal (cartilage or skeletal muscle) forms.[113,114] They usually present with androgenic manifestations or symptoms of a pelvic mass (solid or solid cystic, less frequently cystic), but also can have estrogenic manifestations. Average age at presentation is 25 years with a wide range (1–84 years); those with a retiform morphology tend to occur in younger patients, whereas they are well-differentiated in older patients. SLCT has been reported in the setting of DICER1 syndrome.[103,115,116] Usually, these patients have a germline loss-of-function mutation and a somatic hotspot mutation in their tumors as a second hit. The risk of having a germline *DICER1* mutation after a diagnosis of ovarian SLCT can be as high as 69%.[117,118] In addition, this syndrome has low penetrance and, therefore, the lack of a family history or lack of other DICER1 syndrome related tumors in the patient might be misleading. Taken together, it is recommended that any woman with an SLCT should receive genetic counseling for DICER1 syndrome, unless screening for *DICER1* mutation in the tumor is possible as a first line approach (in which case, a negative result is reassuring, but a positive result should be followed by germline testing).

Box 3
Molecular pathology features: pure sex cord tumors

Adult granulosa cell tumor, somatic alterations:
- Most common (usually ≥90%): *FOXL2* c.C402G (p.C134W) mutation
- High-grade transformation: *TP53* mutations
- Recurrent: Predominantly *TERT* promoter mutations; however, *KMT2D* (seen in approximately 10% of AGCT), *TP53*, and *MED12* mutations, and *CDKN2A/B* homozygous deletions also anecdotally observed

Juvenile granulosa cell tumor
- Somatic: Commonly *AKT1*, *GNAS*, *KMT2C*, *TERT* rearrangements, *DICER1*; rarely *IDH1* and *FOXL2*
- Syndromic: Ollier (*IDH1*), Mafucci (*IDH1*), DICER1 syndrome

---

Box 4
Differential diagnosis: pure sex cord tumors

Adult granulosa cell tumor
- Fibrothecomatous tumors: Reticulin around individual cells
- Endometrioid carcinoma: EMA+
- FOXL2 immunostain: Not a surrogate for the mutation, but can be used for SCST lineage confirmation (also positive in other SCSTs)
- *FOXL2* mutation testing: Relatively sensitive and specific, but not definitive (particularly if differential includes SLCT in a postmenopausal women)

Juvenile granulosa cell tumor
- Small cell carcinoma, hypercalcemic type: Follicle-like spaces lined by small blue cells that lack polarization, EMA+, SMARCA4 lost
- Yolk sac tumor: Schiller Duval bodies, SALL4+

DICER1 mutations are common in SLCTs with moderate to poor differentiation.[117] Overall, they are present in approximately 65% of SLCTs,[9,108,109,117–121] a frequency that is slightly skewed upwards because of the studies with subject populations enriched in patients with DICER1 syndrome (up to 97%).[118] Recently, a more inclusive study in terms of patient demographics has proposed that SLCTs have 3 molecular subgroups correlating with their clinicopathologic features[122]: *DICER1* (44%), *FOXL2* (19%), and non-*DICER1/FOXL2* (37%) mutated (**Fig. 6**, **Box 5**). Those with *DICER1* mutations were seen in the younger patients (median age, 24.5 years), whereas *FOXL2* occurs in older patients (median age, 79.5 years) and those wild type for both in between (median age, 51 years). *DICER1*-mutated cases had the typical clinical and morphologic features of SLCT with predominantly androgenic symptoms and moderate to poor differentiation, as well as the presence of heterologous and retiform elements. In contrast, *FOXL2*-mutated ones were seen in postmenopausal patients with abnormal bleeding, which also had moderate to poor differentiation, but without heterologous elements. Of note, the authors performed a thorough morphologic assessment to make sure these did not represent luteinized AGCTs. In addition, another study simultaneously also described *FOXL2* mutations in an SLCT,[23] supportive the concept of a *FOXL2*-mutated SLCT category. The third group (*FOXL2* and *DICER1* wild type) mostly included well-differentiated SLCTs. The prognostic significance of this classification is currently unclear owing to the limited number of cases; however, it still has immediate implications for genetic counseling in the setting of DICER1 syndrome (which should be considered at least in all SLCT of intermediate or poor differentiation, particularly if retiform or heterologous components are found).

Most of the mimickers of SLCTs are usually discernible by morphologic features (**Fig. 7**) with occasional help from ancillary studies. Among them, perhaps the most challenging one would be the differentiation of a luteinized AGCT from a *FOXL2*-mutated SLCT without heterologous elements, as ancillary testing including mutational profile would not be useful. Morphologically, SLCT usually does not have a fibromatous stroma like AGCT, and rather has a lobulated architecture in an edematous stroma. The Leydig cells usually are clustered at the periphery of the sertoliform lobules, whereas in AGCT the luteinized cells are scattered throughout the stroma usually in a single-cell manner (see **Fig. 7**C, D). However, especially after *FOXL2* mutation status is established, perhaps the distinction of these 2 entities is of uncertain clinical significance. Overall, the similar clinical presentation and mutation profiles may indicate a spectrum of the same pathophysiology and additional studies are warranted.

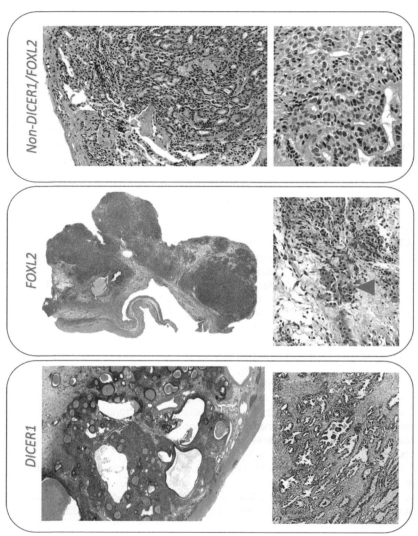

Fig. 6. Typical morphologic characteristics of the molecular SLCT subgroups. *DICER1*-mutated: Intermediate differentiation with heterologous elements in the form of intestinal epithelium (*top*). Retiform architecture mimicking rete testis (*bottom*). *FOXL2*-mutated: intermediate differentiation with lobulated architecture and without heterologous elements (*top*). Leydig cell clusters (arrowhead) at the periphery of the nodules (*bottom*). Non-*DICER1/FOXL2* mutated: well-differentiated SLCT (*top*). Leydig cells intermixed with the well-formed tubules (*bottom*).

Box 5
Molecular pathology features: Sertoli-Leydig cell tumors

DICER1-mutated
- If syndromic: Germline loss of function + somatic hotspot mutations
- Nonsyndromic: Usually somatic hotspot mutations
- Younger patients (mean, 24.5 years; range, 15–62 years)
- Androgenic manifestations
- Intermediate to poorly differentiated histology
- Retiform or heterologous elements common
- *DICER1* somatic alterations can be used to differentiate from AGCT

FOXL2-mutated
- Older patients (mean, 79.5 years; range, 51–90 years)
- Estrogenic > androgenic manifestations
- Intermediate to poorly differentiated histology
- No retiform or heterologous elements
- Distinction from AGCT should be done based on morphology

DICER1 and *FOXL2* wild type
- Intermediate age (mean 51, years; range, 17–74 years)
- Includes well-differentiated SLCTs

Clinics Care Points

- Currently, any woman with a diagnosis of ovarian SLCT should be considered for genetic counseling for DICER1 syndrome.
- In an ideal scenario, an initial screening of tumor DNA for *DICER1* alterations can eliminate *DICER1*-wild type cases and capture the high-risk population of *DICER1*-mutated tumors for genetic counseling.

Sex Cord–Stromal Tumor, Not Otherwise Specified and Gynandroblastoma

SCST, not otherwise specified, does not have any definitive characteristic of a specific SCST category (pure stromal, pure sex cord, or SLCT as listed in **Tables 1** and **2**), but has a morphologic and immunohistochemical clues of a sex cord-stromal lineage.[10] A recent series of challenging SCSTs showed that molecular analysis for *FOXL2*, *DICER1*, and *STK11* can help with the diagnosis in approximately 85% of the cases (42/50).[8] Another smaller series had 30% (6/20) of the cases resolved as AGCT based on *FOXL2* analysis.[32] These studies highlight the usefulness of molecular studies in the classification of morphologically-ambiguous SCSTs (**Box 6**).

Gynandroblastomas are presumed mixed tumors with components resembling both female (gyn-) and male (andro-) sex cord differentiation with varying stromal elements,[1,123] with an arbitrary cut off of having at least 10% of each morphology.[124] Overall, they are relatively indolent with only 2 recurrences in the literature.[125,126] Historically, SCST, not otherwise specified, and gynandroblastomas have been recognized as 2 different entities; however, in practice it may be difficult to make a definitive distinction depending on the percentage of each morphology and presence of their defining features. Not surprisingly, both terms have been used for tumors having overlapping characteristics in the literature. An additional challenge is to discern a true mixed SCST with collision of different tumor types from a rare morphologic variant of a single entity having areas resembling to another SCST. Given the rarity of these scenarios, currently it is difficult to speculate the clinical significance of separating or further defining SCST, not otherwise specified, from gynandroblastoma. For now, a clear and consistent nomenclature should be followed as much as possible for future

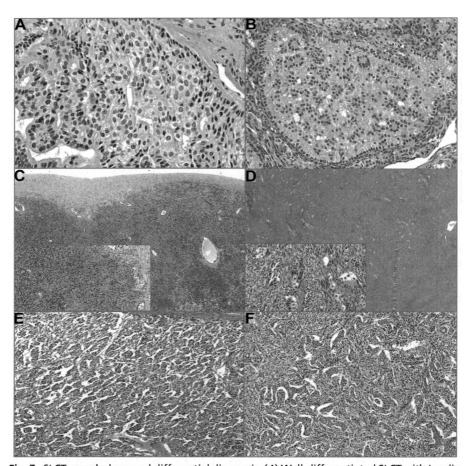

Fig. 7. SLCT morphology and differential diagnosis. (*A*) Well-differentiated SLCT with Leydig cells intermixed with sertoliform tubules. (*B*) Sex cord tumor with annular tubules with anti-polar distribution of nuclei around basement membrane-like material. (*C*) SLCT with inter-mediate differentiation (*inset*, clusters of Leydig cells prominent at the periphery of the lobules). (*D*) AGCT with luteinization and fibromatous stroma (*inset*, scattered lutein cells throughout the stroma). (*E*) Retiform SLCT with somewhat papillary configuration of the Sertoli cells. (*F*) AGCT forming a trabeculated architecture with peculiar clefting mimicking the small papillae seen in retiform SLCT.

accumulation of data and better stratification of patients. Of note, the subcategories discussed in the following paragraphs are not included in the 2020 World Health Or-ganization classification[10] and are only used for better organization of the existing literature.

Tumors with Sertoli and Adult Granulosa Morphology

A single study looking at individual components of gynandroblastomas[127] showed that *FOXL2* or *DICER1* mutations were absent in all tumors with adult granulosa morphology with an accompanying Sertoli cell morphology (6/6).[127] It was interesting to note the majority of these cases had a well-differentiated Sertoli component (**Fig. 8**).

Box 6
Molecular pathology features: SCST not otherwise specified and gynandroblastoma

- Tumors with overlapping fibrothecomatous and adult granulosa cell morphology are difficult to classify morphologically. A reticulin stain and/or *FOXL2* mutation testing can be extremely helpful in this setting.

- Tumors with Sertoli and JGCT-like morphology may represent a morphologic variant of *DICER1*-mutated SLCTs with juvenile granulosa-like differentiation.

- Tumors with adult granulosa cell and well-differentiated Sertoli morphology seem to be most frequently *DICER1*-and *FOXL2*-wild type, linking them with the group of SLCTs that is also well differentiated and lacks mutations in these genes.

- Tumors with true biphasic morphology may exist (gynandroblastomas and true collision tumors); however, at least some gynandroblastomas have been shown to be tumors with morphologic ambiguity mimicking a collision phenomenon and have been re-classified as a specific SCST entity (for instance, SLCT with JGCT-like growth).

In fact, none of the gynandroblastomas with well-differentiated Sertoli morphology in this study (7/7) showed either *FOXL2* or *DICER1* mutations, akin to the *FOXL2* and *DICER1* wild-type SLCTs that are enriched in well-differentiated morphology.[122] Another study with 3 tumors with Sertoli cell and AGCT morphology also had wild

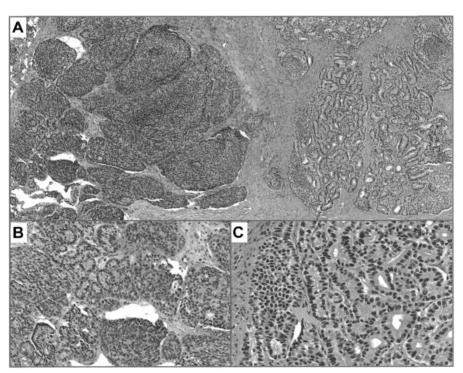

Fig. 8. (*A*) Tumor with adult granulosa (*left*) and well-differentiated Sertoli cell (*right*) morphology. (*B*) Sertoliform tubules intermixed with the adult granulosa background. (*C*) Well-differentiated Sertoli cell tubules transitioning into adult granulosa-like areas (*arrow*).

type *FOXL2* in either component.[128] Another case of an AGCT and sex cord stromal tumor with annular tubules morphologies did not demonstrate either *DICER1* or *FOXL2* mutations.[8] In addition, the previously mentioned consult series of AGCTs with 70% *FOXL2* mutations[78] pointed out that many of the *FOXL2*-wild type cases had additional sex cord-stromal components. Overall, these findings indicate that the small subset of *FOXL2*-negative AGCTs are often enriched in other sex cord elements and suggest that they may have a morphologic and presumably undiscovered molecular continuum with FOXL2/*DICER1*-wild type well-differentiated SLCT that may occasionally mimic a mixed tumor (see **Fig. 8**). Additional studies analyzing the clonality of each component for other molecular markers maybe of interest to support this hypothesis.

Tumors with Sertoli Cell and Juvenile Granulosa Morphology

The previously mentioned study looking at individual components of gynandroblastomas[127] reported 40% (3/8) of tumors with moderate to poorly differentiated Sertoli cell component showed *DICER1* mutations, all of which also had additional juvenile granulosa morphology also showing the same mutations. Although this is the only report with the analysis of each component, multiple additional studies documented moderate to poorly differentiated Sertoli cell with juvenile granulosa morphology (the majority of them referred to as gynandroblastomas) having *DICER1* alterations,[110,117,121] including those seen in patients with DICER1 syndrome.[117,118,126] As mentioned previously in this article, *DICER1* relatively are a hallmark change in SLCT, and are in turn rare in JGCT. In addition, a recent study showed that SLCTs with JGCT-like follicles have (1) clinical features more akin to SLCT rather than JGCT, and (2) a predominant SLCT morphology where JGCT-like follicles gradually arise from the lobules of SLCT (**Fig. 9**).[129] Overall, these findings suggest that so-called gynandroblastomas with Sertoli cell and juvenile granulosa morphology likely represent a morphologic variant of *DICER1*-mutated SLCTs that shows JGCT-like differentiation and the subset of JGCTs with *DICER1* mutations may represent a continuum of these tumors.

An alternative but rare consideration in this morphologic spectrum is the high-grade transformation of an SLCT, which is exemplified by a single case of SLCT demonstrating *DICER1* and *TP53* mutations,[8] akin to the AGCTs with high-grade transformation having *FOXL2* and *TP53* mutations.

Tumors with Adult and Juvenile Granulosa Morphology

Other than personal anecdotes of expert pathologists, there is only a single example of a combined AGCT and JGCT in the literature, which also has a Sertoli cell tumor component.[130] However, the authors of the AGCT with high-grade differentiation study[93] made a valid point in their discussion that perhaps a subset of these can be misinterpreted as mixed SCST with AGCT and JGCT components owing to pleomorphic and focally cystic morphology of the high-grade component. The authors of this study found *FOXL2* mutations in both AGCT and high-grade components, excluding this possibility and, in turn, suggesting a common clonal origin of the AGCT with JGCT-like elements in those cases with high-grade transformation.

Fibrothecomatous Tumors with Adult Granulosa Morphology (So-Called Granulosa–Theca Cell Tumors)

Fibrothecomatous tumors with less than 10% sex cord elements have been referred to as stromal tumors with minor sex cord elements, and they are considered benign in nature.[132] Some pathologists use the term granulosa-theca cell tumors for those with 10% to 50% granulosa cells in a fibrothecomatous background,[34,35] whereas

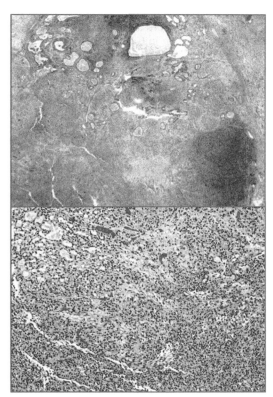

Fig. 9. SLCT with juvenile granulosa-like follicular differentiation: Follicles arising from the SLCT of intermediate differentiation lobules (*top*) and loosening of the pale stroma yielding to follicle-like structures (*bottom*).

others call any tumor with a granulosa component beyond 10% as AGCTs. When called AGCTs, these tumors will be in the spectrum of AGCTs with thecoma-like foci and AGCT with extensive fibromatous background (see **Figs. 1**E,F and **4**C, D).

In the previously mentioned series of challenging SCSTs,[8] the most common dilemma (29/50) was AGCTs with overlapping features with thecomas and cellular fibromas (and an additional cystic AGCT with a differential diagnosis of follicle cyst not included in this discussion but characterized further in a recent series[131]). Given that reticulin is not always conclusive,[23] *FOXL2* mutation analysis can be more sensitive in this setting. In this study, 15 of 29 tumors with the above differential were classified as AGCT based on morphologic features and the presence of *FOXL2* mutation, whereas only 1 in 29 cases was diagnosed as an AGCT despite the lack of *FOXL2* mutation based on morphologic clues only. In contrast, 13 of the 29 tumors were diagnosed as thecoma or cellular fibroma due to lack of *FOXL2* mutation. Overall, *FOXL2* mutation testing was helpful in 28 of the 29 cases with this differential, where only in one AGCT the authors deferred to the morphologic impression, despite the lack of *FOXL2* mutation. Four of these 29 cases had minor sex cord elements. Among those, only one had a *FOXL2* mutation and was therefore reassigned as an AGCT. Of interest, this case had a fibromathecomatous background; therefore, the AGCT component might have been underestimated. Related to this point, in a separate small series, 3 ovarian fibromas with minor sex cord elements were not found to have the *FOXL2* mutation,[25] which is supportive of the overall benign notion of these cases.

A separate study documenting tumors classified as granulosa theca cell tumors of the ovary[36] reported *FOXL2* mutation in 6 of 12 tumors. The mutation was found in both fibromathecomatous and granulosa components in all 5 of 6 *FOXL2*-positive tumors that underwent microdissection and sequencing of both components. This finding may be analogous to the morphologic illusion seen in the AGCT with thecoma-like foci, where even though on the hematoxylin and eosin staining alone the classic morphology is limited (see **Fig. 1E**), reticulin stain highlights the majority of the tumor nodules being nested (see **Fig. 1F**). This phenomenon is important because it may cause underestimation of the AGCT component based on morphology alone. Overall, the data presented herein further question the existence of thecomas with *FOXL2* mutations. Particularly in the setting of a previously discussed example of a thecoma with a *FOXL2* mutation relapsing in 2 years with a classical AGCT morphology,[31] perhaps any thecoma with a *FOXL2* mutation should be interpreted with caution regarding their malignancy potential.

Collision Tumor

A true collision tumor with both morphologic and molecular evidence is extremely rare to come across among these exceedingly rare tumors. However, there is at least one example in the literature describing a steroid cell tumor and SRST in the same ovary,[64] with only the latter tumor having a beta catenin nuclear localization. In addition, the 2 morphologies seemed to have an abrupt change without any intermingling between the 2 components. Therefore, in this particular case, the morphologic and molecular features suggest different clonality of each component in keeping with a collision tumor. Of note, as previously discussed, the SRST in this tumor may represent a nonconventional MST (see **Fig. 3D**) based on the provided image. Currently, this distinction is difficult to make and requires further studies for a more definitive categorization.

CLINICS CARE POINTS

- Reticulin staining and *FOXL2* mutation analysis are helpful diagnostic tools in separating AGCTs from thecomas with nodular morphology and mitotically active cellular fibromas.

- *FOXL2* and *TERT* promoter mutations can be detected as biomarkers in cell-free AGCT DNA for disease monitoring.

- Sex cord–stromal tumor, not otherwise specified, diagnoses can further be screened for *DICER1*, *FOXL2*, and/or *STK11* mutation status depending on the scenario for better categorization of these tumors.

- Molecular subtypes of SLCTs (*FOXL2*, *DICER1*, non-*FOXL2/DICER1*) have overlap in clinical presentation and molecular features with AGCTs (*FOXL2*, as well as non-*FOXL2/DICER1*), JGCTs (*DICER1*), and so-called gynandroblastomas (*DICER1*, as well as non-*FOXL2/DICER1*).

- The diagnosis of an SLCT should prompt genetic counseling, given that tumor *DICER1* mutation testing is not routinely offered, *DICER1* syndrome has low penetrance and therefore, lack of personal and family history of *DICER1* related tumors may be misleading.

ACKNOWLEDGMENTS

The author thanks to Dr Robert Henry Young for sharing his consultation files, which were used for the majority of the photomicrographs herein and Dr McCluggage for providing the nonconventional MST image.

DISCLOSURE

The author has no disclosures to make.

REFERENCES

1. Morris JM, Scully RE. Endocrine pathology of the ovary. St. Louis: The C. V. Mosby Company; 1958.
2. Young RH. Ovarian sex cord-stromal tumors: reflections on a 40-year experience with a fascinating group of tumors, including comments on the seminal observations of Robert E. Scully, MD. Arch Pathol Lab Med 2018;142(12):1459–84.
3. Young RH. Ovarian sex cord-stromal tumours and their mimics. Pathology 2018; 50(1):5–15.
4. Hanley KZ, Mosunjac MB. Practical Review of Ovarian Sex Cord-Stromal Tumors. Surg Pathol Clin 2019;12(2):587–620.
5. McCluggage WG, Young RH. Immunohistochemistry as a diagnostic aid in the evaluation of ovarian tumors. Semin Diagn Pathol 2005;22(1):3–32.
6. Rabban JT, Zaloudek CJ. A practical approach to immunohistochemical diagnosis of ovarian germ cell tumours and sex cord-stromal tumours. Histopathology 2013;62(1):71–88.
7. Lim D, Oliva E. Ovarian sex cord-stromal tumours: an update in recent molecular advances. Pathology 2018;50(2):178–89.
8. Stewart CJR, Amanuel B, De Kock L, et al. Evaluation of molecular analysis in challenging ovarian sex cord-stromal tumours: a review of 50 cases. Pathology 2020;52(6):686–93.
9. Rabban JT, Karnezis AN, Devine WP. Practical roles for molecular diagnostic testing in ovarian adult granulosa cell tumour, Sertoli-Leydig cell tumour, microcystic stromal tumour and their mimics. Histopathology 2020;76(1):11–24.
10. WHO classification of tumours: female genital tumours. 5th edition. vol. 4. Lyon (France): International Agency for Research on Cancer; 2020.
11. Prat J, Scully RE. Cellular fibromas and fibrosarcomas of the ovary: a comparative clinicopathologic analysis of seventeen cases. Cancer 1981;47(11): 2663–70.
12. Meigs JV. Fibroma of the ovary with ascites and hydrothorax; Meigs' syndrome. Am J Obstet Gynecol 1954;67(5):962–85.
13. Gorlin RJ. Nevoid basal-cell carcinoma syndrome. Medicine (Baltimore) 1987; 66(2):98–113.
14. Evans DG, Oudit D, Smith MJ, et al. First evidence of genotype-phenotype correlations in Gorlin syndrome. J Med Genet 2017;54(8):530–6.
15. Kenny SL, Patel K, Humphries A, et al. Ovarian cellular fibroma harbouring an isocitrate dehydrogenase 1 (1DH1) mutation in a patient with Ollier disease: evidence for a causal relationship. Histopathology 2013;62(4):667–70.
16. Shashi V, Golden WL, von Kap-Herr C, et al. Interphase fluorescence in situ hybridization for trisomy 12 on archival ovarian sex cord-stromal tumors. Gynecol Oncol 1994;55(3 Pt 1):349–54.
17. Tsuji T, Kawauchi S, Utsunomiya T, et al. Fibrosarcoma versus cellular fibroma of the ovary: a comparative study of their proliferative activity and chromosome aberrations using MIB-1 immunostaining, DNA flow cytometry, and fluorescence in situ hybridization. Am J Surg Pathol 1997;21(1):52–9.
18. Kato N, Romero M, Catasus L, et al. The STK11/LKB1 Peutz-Jegher gene is not involved in the pathogenesis of sporadic sex cord-stromal tumors, although loss

of heterozygosity at 19p13.3 indicates other gene alteration in these tumors. Hum Pathol 2004;35(9):1101–4.

19. Tsuji T, Catasus L, Prat J. Is loss of heterozygosity at 9q22.3 (PTCH gene) and 19p13.3 (STK11 gene) involved in the pathogenesis of ovarian stromal tumors? Hum Pathol 2005;36(7):792–6.

20. Streblow RC, Dafferner AJ, Nelson M, et al. Imbalances of chromosomes 4, 9, and 12 are recurrent in the thecoma-fibroma group of ovarian stromal tumors. Cancer Genet Cytogenet 2007;178(2):135–40.

21. Hunter SM, Dall GV, Doyle MA, et al. Molecular comparison of pure ovarian fibroma with serous benign ovarian tumours. BMC Res Notes 2020;13(1):349.

22. Irving JA, Alkushi A, Young RH, et al. Cellular fibromas of the ovary: a study of 75 cases including 40 mitotically active tumors emphasizing their distinction from fibrosarcoma. Am J Surg Pathol 2006;30(8):929–38.

23. Buza N, Wong S, Hui P. FOXL2 mutation analysis of ovarian sex cord-stromal tumors: genotype-phenotype correlation with diagnostic considerations. Int J Gynecol Pathol 2018;37(4):305–15.

24. Shah SP, Kobel M, Senz J, et al. Mutation of FOXL2 in granulosa-cell tumors of the ovary. N Engl J Med 2009;360(26):2719–29.

25. McCluggage WG, Singh N, Kommoss S, et al. Ovarian cellular fibromas lack FOXL2 mutations: a useful diagnostic adjunct in the distinction from diffuse adult granulosa cell tumor. Am J Surg Pathol 2013;37(9):1450–5.

26. Loeffler EP A. Bindegewebige Gewächse des Eierstockes von besonderer Bauart (Fibroma thecocellulare xanthomatodes ovarii). Beitr Path Anat 1932; 90:199–221.

27. Burandt E, Young RH. Thecoma of the ovary: a report of 70 cases emphasizing aspects of its histopathology different from those often portrayed and its differential diagnosis. Am J Surg Pathol 2014;38(8):1023–32.

28. Bjorkholm E, Silfversward C. Theca-cell tumors. Clinical features and prognosis. Acta Radiol Oncol 1980;19(4):241–4.

29. Young RH, Clement PB, Scully RE. Calcified thecomas in young women. A report of four cases. Int J Gynecol Pathol 1988;7(4):343–50.

30. Kim MS, Hur SY, Yoo NJ, et al. Mutational analysis of FOXL2 codon 134 in granulosa cell tumour of ovary and other human cancers. J Pathol 2010;221(2): 147–52.

31. Al-Agha OM, Huwait HF, Chow C, et al. FOXL2 is a sensitive and specific marker for sex cord-stromal tumors of the ovary. Am J Surg Pathol 2011;35(4):484–94.

32. Kommoss S, Anglesio MS, Mackenzie R, et al. FOXL2 molecular testing in ovarian neoplasms: diagnostic approach and procedural guidelines. Mod Pathol 2013;26(6):860–7.

33. Stall JN, Young RH. Granulosa cell tumors of the ovary with prominent thecoma-like foci: a report of 16 cases emphasizing the ongoing utility of the reticulin stain in the modern era. Int J Gynecol Pathol 2019;38(2):143–50.

34. Stage AH, Grafton WD. Thecomas and granulosa-theca cell tumors of the ovary: an analysis of 51 tumors. Obstet Gynecol 1977;50(1):21–7.

35. Norris HJ, Taylor HB. Prognosis of granulosa-theca tumors of the ovary. Cancer 1968;21(2):255–63.

36. Nolan A, Joseph NM, Sangoi AR, et al. FOXL2 mutation status in granulosa theca cell tumors of the ovary. Int J Gynecol Pathol 2017;36(6):568–74.

37. Chalvardjian A, Scully RE. Sclerosing stromal tumors of the ovary. Cancer 1973; 31(3):664–70.

38. Devins KM, Young RH, Watkins JC. Sclerosing stromal tumour: a clinicopathological study of 100 cases of a distinctive benign ovarian stromal tumour typically occurring in the young. Histopathology 2021. https://doi.org/10.1111/his.14554.

39. Bennett JA, Oliva E, Young RH. Sclerosing stromal tumors with prominent luteinization during pregnancy: a report of 8 cases emphasizing diagnostic problems. Int J Gynecol Pathol 2015;34(4):357–62.

40. Goebel EA, McCluggage WG, Walsh JC. Mitotically active sclerosing stromal tumor of the ovary: report of a case series with parallels to mitotically active cellular fibroma. Int J Gynecol Pathol 2016;35(6):549–53.

41. Grechi G, Clemente N, Tozzi A, et al. Laparoscopic treatment of sclerosing stromal tumor of the ovary in a woman with Gorlin-Goltz syndrome: a case report and review of the literature. J Minim Invasive Gynecol 2015;22(5):892–5.

42. Kostopoulou E, Moulla A, Giakoustidis D, et al. Sclerosing stromal tumors of the ovary: a clinicopathologic, immunohistochemical and cytogenetic analysis of three cases. Eur J Gynaecol Oncol 2004;25(2):257–60.

43. Kawauchi S, Tsuji T, Kaku T, et al. Sclerosing stromal tumor of the ovary: a clinicopathologic, immunohistochemical, ultrastructural, and cytogenetic analysis with special reference to its vasculature. Am J Surg Pathol 1998;22(1):83–92.

44. Kim SH, Da Cruz Paula A, Basili T, et al. Identification of recurrent FHL2-GLI2 oncogenic fusion in sclerosing stromal tumors of the ovary. Nat Commun 2020;11(1):44.

45. Devins KM, Young RH, Croce S, et al. Solitary fibrous tumors of the female genital tract: a study of 27 cases emphasizing nonvulvar locations, variant histology, and prognostic factors. Am J Surg Pathol 2021;8. https://doi.org/10.1097/PAS.0000000000001829.

46. Yang EJ, Howitt BE, Fletcher CDM, et al. Solitary fibrous tumour of the female genital tract: a clinicopathological analysis of 25 cases. Histopathology 2018;72(5):749–59.

47. Irving JA, Young RH. Microcystic stromal tumor of the ovary: report of 16 cases of a hitherto uncharacterized distinctive ovarian neoplasm. Am J Surg Pathol 2009;33(3):367–75.

48. McCluggage WG, Chong AS, Attygalle AD, et al. Expanding the morphological spectrum of ovarian microcystic stromal tumour. Histopathology 2019;74(3):443–51.

49. Parra-Herran C, McCluggage WG. Ovarian microcystic stromal tumour: from morphological observations to syndromic associations. Histopathology. 2022 Jan 12. https://doi.org/10.1111/his.14616. Epub ahead of print. PMID: 35020947.

50. Parra-Herran C. Endometrioid tubal intraepithelial neoplasia and bilateral ovarian microcystic stromal tumors harboring APC mutations: report of a case. Int J Gynecol Pathol 2021. https://doi.org/10.1097/PGP.0000000000000814.

51. Lee SH, Koh YW, Roh HJ, et al. Ovarian microcystic stromal tumor: a novel extracolonic tumor in familial adenomatous polyposis. Genes Chromosomes Cancer 2015;54(6):353–60.

52. McCluggage WG, Irving JA, Chong AS, et al. Ovarian microcystic stromal tumors are characterized by alterations in the beta-catenin-APC pathway and may be an extracolonic manifestation of familial adenomatous polyposis. Am J Surg Pathol 2018;42(1):137–9.

53. Maeda D, Shibahara J, Sakuma T, et al. beta-catenin (CTNNB1) S33C mutation in ovarian microcystic stromal tumors. Am J Surg Pathol 2011;35(10):1429–40.

54. Irving JA, Lee CH, Yip S, et al. Microcystic Stromal Tumor: A Distinctive Ovarian Sex Cord-Stromal Neoplasm Characterized by FOXL2, SF-1, WT-1, Cyclin D1, and beta-catenin Nuclear Expression and CTNNB1 Mutations. Am J Surg Pathol 2015;39(10):1420–6.

55. Bi R, Bai QM, Yang F, et al. Microcystic stromal tumour of the ovary: frequent mutations of beta-catenin (CTNNB1) in six cases. Histopathology 2015;67(6):872–9.

56. Meurgey A, Descotes F, Mery-Lamarche E, et al. Lack of mutation of DICER1 and FOXL2 genes in microcystic stromal tumor of the ovary. Virchows Arch 2017;470(2):225–9.

57. Zhang Y, Tao L, Yin C, et al. Ovarian microcystic stromal tumor with undetermined potential: case study with molecular analysis and literature review. Hum Pathol 2018;78:171–6.

58. Man X, Wei Z, Wang B, et al. Ovarian microcystic stromal tumor with omental metastasis: the first case report and literature review. J Ovarian Res 2021;14(1):73.

59. Ramzy I. Signet-ring stromal tumor of ovary. Histochemical, light, and electron microscopic study. Cancer 1976;38(1):166–72.

60. Dickersin GR, Young RH, Scully RE. Signet-ring stromal and related tumors of the ovary. Ultrastruct Pathol 1995;19(5):401–19.

61. Vang R, Bague S, Tavassoli FA, et al. Signet-ring stromal tumor of the ovary: clinicopathologic analysis and comparison with Krukenberg tumor. Int J Gynecol Pathol 2004;23(1):45–51.

62. Michalova K, Michal M Jr, Kazakov DV, et al. Primary signet ring stromal tumor of the testis: a study of 13 cases indicating their phenotypic and genotypic analogy to pancreatic solid pseudopapillary neoplasm. Hum Pathol 2017;67:85–93.

63. Kopczynski J, Kowalik A, Chlopek M, et al. Oncogenic activation of the Wnt/beta-catenin signaling pathway in signet ring stromal cell tumor of the ovary. Appl Immunohistochem Mol Morphol 2016;24(5):e28–33.

64. McGregor SM, Schoolmeester JK, Lastra RR. Collision signet-ring stromal tumor and steroid cell tumor of the ovary: report of the first case. Int J Gynecol Pathol 2017;36(3):261–4.

65. Chen PH, Hui P, Buza N. Bilateral signet-ring stromal tumor of the ovary: a case report with next-generation sequencing analysis and FOXL2 mutation testing. Int J Gynecol Pathol 2020;39(2):193–8.

66. Deshpande V, Oliva E, Young RH. Solid pseudopapillary neoplasm of the ovary: a report of 3 primary ovarian tumors resembling those of the pancreas. Am J Surg Pathol 2010;34(10):1514–20.

67. Singh K, Patel N, Patil P, et al. Primary ovarian solid pseudopapillary neoplasm with CTNNB1 c.98C>G (p.S33C) point mutation. Int J Gynecol Pathol 2018;37(2):110–6.

68. Choi Y, Choi H, Kim HS, et al. Signet-ring stromal cell tumour of the ovary confused with Krukenberg's tumour; a case report. J Obstet Gynaecol 2021;41(1):155–7.

69. Kiyokawa T, Young RH, Scully RE. Krukenberg tumors of the ovary: a clinicopathologic analysis of 120 cases with emphasis on their variable pathologic manifestations. Am J Surg Pathol 2006;30(3):277–99.

70. Bennett JA, Young RH, Chuang AY, et al. Ovarian metastases of breast cancers with signet ring cells: a report of 17 cases including 14 Krukenberg tumors. Int J Gynecol Pathol 2018;37(6):507–15.
71. Hu PJ, Knoepp SM, Wu R, et al. Ovarian steroid cell tumor with biallelic adenomatous polyposis coli inactivation in a patient with familial adenomatous polyposis. Genes Chromosomes Cancer 2012;51(3):283–9.
72. Lee IH, Choi CH, Hong DG, et al. Clinicopathologic characteristics of granulosa cell tumors of the ovary: a multicenter retrospective study. J Gynecol Oncol 2011;22(3):188–95.
73. Nogales FF, Musto ML, Saez AI, et al. Multifocal intrafollicular granulosa cell tumor of the ovary associated with an unusual germline p53 mutation. Mod Pathol 2004;17(7):868–73.
74. Jamieson S, Butzow R, Andersson N, et al. The FOXL2 C134W mutation is characteristic of adult granulosa cell tumors of the ovary. Mod Pathol 2010;23(11):1477–85.
75. Kim T, Sung CO, Song SY, et al. FOXL2 mutation in granulosa-cell tumours of the ovary. Histopathology 2010;56(3):408–10.
76. Roze J, Monroe G, Kutzera J, et al. Whole genome analysis of ovarian granulosa cell tumors reveals tumor heterogeneity and a high-grade TP53-specific subgroup. Cancers (Basel) 2020;12(5):1308.
77. Oseto K, Suzumori N, Nishikawa R, et al. Mutational analysis of FOXL2 p.C134W and expression of bone morphogenetic protein 2 in Japanese patients with granulosa cell tumor of ovary. J Obstet Gynaecol Res 2014;40(5):1197–204.
78. D'Angelo E, Mozos A, Nakayama D, et al. Prognostic significance of FOXL2 mutation and mRNA expression in adult and juvenile granulosa cell tumors of the ovary. Mod Pathol 2011;24(10):1360–7.
79. Rosario R, Wilson M, Cheng WT, et al. Adult granulosa cell tumours (GCT): clinicopathological outcomes including FOXL2 mutational status and expression. Gynecol Oncol 2013;131(2):325–9.
80. Caburet S, Georges A, L'Hote D, et al. The transcription factor FOXL2: at the crossroads of ovarian physiology and pathology. Mol Cell Endocrinol 2012;356(1–2):55–64.
81. Crisponi L, Deiana M, Loi A, et al. The putative forkhead transcription factor FOXL2 is mutated in blepharophimosis/ptosis/epicanthus inversus syndrome. Nat Genet 2001;27(2):159–66.
82. Pilsworth JA, Todeschini AL, Neilson SJ, et al. FOXL2 in adult-type granulosa cell tumour of the ovary: oncogene or tumour suppressor gene? J Pathol 2021;255(3):225–31.
83. Mangili G, Ottolina J, Gadducci A, et al. Long-term follow-up is crucial after treatment for granulosa cell tumours of the ovary. Br J Cancer 2013;109(1):29–34.
84. Miller K, McCluggage WG. Prognostic factors in ovarian adult granulosa cell tumour. J Clin Pathol 2008;61(8):881–4.
85. Sun HD, Lin H, Jao MS, et al. A long-term follow-up study of 176 cases with adult-type ovarian granulosa cell tumors. Gynecol Oncol 2012;124(2):244–9.
86. Pilsworth JA, Cochrane DR, Xia Z, et al. TERT promoter mutation in adult granulosa cell tumor of the ovary. Mod Pathol 2018;31(7):1107–15.
87. Alexiadis M, Rowley SM, Chu S, et al. Mutational landscape of ovarian adult granulosa cell tumors from whole exome and targeted TERT promoter sequencing. Mol Cancer Res 2019;17(1):177–85.

88. Da Cruz Paula A, da Silva EM, Segura SE, et al. Genomic profiling of primary and recurrent adult granulosa cell tumors of the ovary. Mod Pathol 2020; 33(8):1606–17.

89. Groeneweg JW, Roze JF, Peters EDJ, et al. FOXL2 and TERT promoter mutation detection in circulating tumor DNA of adult granulosa cell tumors as biomarker for disease monitoring. Gynecol Oncol 2021;162(2):413–20.

90. Farkkila A, McConechy MK, Yang W, et al. FOXL2 402C>G mutation can be identified in the circulating tumor DNA of patients with adult-type granulosa cell tumor. J Mol Diagn 2017;19(1):126–36.

91. Pilsworth JA, Cochrane DR, Neilson SJ, et al. Adult-type granulosa cell tumor of the ovary: a FOXL2-centric disease. J Pathol Clin Res 2021;7(3):243–52.

92. Hillman RT, Celestino J, Terranova C, et al. KMT2D/MLL2 inactivation is associated with recurrence in adult-type granulosa cell tumors of the ovary. Nat Commun 2018;9(1):2496.

93. Fashedemi Y, Coutts M, Wise O, et al. Adult granulosa cell tumor with high-grade transformation: report of a series With FOXL2 mutation analysis. Am J Surg Pathol 2019;43(9):1229–38.

94. Mubeen A, Martin I, Dhall D. High-grade Transformation in Adult Granulosa Cell Tumor: Potential Diagnostic Challenges and the Utility of Molecular Testing. Int J Surg Pathol. 2022 Feb 4:10668969221076553. https://doi.org/10.1177/10668969221076553. Epub ahead of print. PMID: 35118890.

95. McNeilage J, Alexiadis M, Susil BJ, et al. Molecular characterization of sarcomatous change in a granulosa cell tumor. Int J Gynecol Cancer 2007;17(2):398–406.

96. Susil BJ, Sumithran E. Sarcomatous change in granulosa cell tumor. Hum Pathol 1987;18(4):397–9.

97. Sonoyama A, Kanda M, Ojima Y, et al. Aggressive granulosa cell tumor of the ovary with rapid recurrence: a case report and review of the literature. Kobe J Med Sci 2015;61(4):E109–14.

98. Young RH, Scully RE. Ovarian sex cord-stromal tumors with bizarre nuclei: a clinicopathologic analysis of 17 cases. Int J Gynecol Pathol 1983;1(4):325–35.

99. Gaffey MJ, Frierson HF Jr, Iezzoni JC, et al. Ovarian granulosa cell tumors with bizarre nuclei: an immunohistochemical analysis with fluorescence in situ hybridization documenting trisomy 12 in the bizarre component [corrected]. Mod Pathol 1996;9(3):308–15.

100. Young RH, Dickersin GR, Scully RE. Juvenile granulosa cell tumor of the ovary. A clinicopathological analysis of 125 cases. Am J Surg Pathol 1984;8(8):575–96.

101. Velasco-Oses A, Alonso-Alvaro A, Blanco-Pozo A, et al. Ollier's disease associated with ovarian juvenile granulosa cell tumor. Cancer 1988;62(1):222–5.

102. Tanaka Y, Sasaki Y, Nishihira H, et al. Ovarian juvenile granulosa cell tumor associated with Maffucci's syndrome. Am J Clin Pathol 1992;97(4):523–7.

103. Schultz KA, Pacheco MC, Yang J, et al. Ovarian sex cord-stromal tumors, pleuropulmonary blastoma and DICER1 mutations: a report from the International Pleuropulmonary Blastoma Registry. Gynecol Oncol 2011;122(2):246–50.

104. Guo H, Keefe KA, Kohler MF, et al. Juvenile granulosa cell tumor of the ovary associated with tuberous sclerosis. Gynecol Oncol 2006;102(1):118–20.

105. Plon SE, Pirics ML, Nuchtern J, et al. Multiple tumors in a child with germ-line mutations in TP53 and PTEN. N Engl J Med 2008;359(5):537–9.

106. Bessiere L, Todeschini AL, Auguste A, et al. A hot-spot of in-frame duplications activates the Oncoprotein AKT1 in juvenile granulosa cell tumors. EBioMedicine 2015;2(5):421–31.

107. Kalfa N, Ecochard A, Patte C, et al. Activating mutations of the stimulatory g protein in juvenile ovarian granulosa cell tumors: a new prognostic factor? J Clin Endocrinol Metab 2006;91(5):1842–7.

108. Heravi-Moussavi A, Anglesio MS, Cheng SW, et al. Recurrent somatic DICER1 mutations in nonepithelial ovarian cancers. N Engl J Med 2012;366(3):234–42.

109. Goulvent T, Ray-Coquard I, Borel S, et al. DICER1 and FOXL2 mutations in ovarian sex cord-stromal tumours: a GINECO Group study. Histopathology 2016;68(2):279–85.

110. Baillard P, Genestie C, Croce S, et al. Rare DICER1 and Absent FOXL2 mutations characterize ovarian juvenile granulosa cell tumors. Am J Surg Pathol 2021;45(2):223–9.

111. Vougiouklakis T, Zhu K, Vasudevaraja V, Serrano J, Shen G, Linn RL, Feng X, Chiang S, Barroeta JE, Thomas KM, Schwartz LE, Shukla PS, Malpica A, Oliva E, Cotzia P, DeLair DF, Snuderl M, Jour G. Integrated Analysis of Ovarian Juvenile Granulosa Cell Tumors Reveals Distinct Epigenetic Signatures and Recurrent *TERT* Rearrangements. Clin Cancer Res. 2022 Jan 14. https://doi.org/10.1158/1078-0432.CCR-21-3394. Epub ahead of print. PMID: 35031544.

112. Young RH, Scully RE. Ovarian Sertoli-Leydig cell tumors. A clinicopathological analysis of 207 cases. Am J Surg Pathol 1985;9(8):543–69.

113. Young RH, Prat J, Scully RE. Ovarian Sertoli-Leydig cell tumors with heterologous elements. I. Gastrointestinal epithelium and carcinoid: a clinicopathologic analysis of thirty-six cases. Cancer 1982;50(11):2448–56.

114. Prat J, Young RH, Scully RE. Ovarian Sertoli-Leydig cell tumors with heterologous elements. II. Cartilage and skeletal muscle: a clinicopathologic analysis of twelve cases. Cancer 1982;50(11):2465–75.

115. Hill DA, Ivanovich J, Priest JR, et al. DICER1 mutations in familial pleuropulmonary blastoma. Science 2009;325(5943):965.

116. Rio Frio T, Bahubeshi A, Kanellopoulou C, et al. DICER1 mutations in familial multinodular goiter with and without ovarian Sertoli-Leydig cell tumors. JAMA 2011;305(1):68–77.

117. de Kock L, Terzic T, McCluggage WG, et al. DICER1 mutations are consistently present in moderately and poorly differentiated Sertoli Leydig cell tumors. Am J Surg Pathol 2017;41(9):1178–87.

118. Schultz KAP, Harris AK, Finch M, et al. DICER1-related Sertoli-Leydig cell tumor and gynandroblastoma: Clinical and genetic findings from the International Ovarian and Testicular Stromal Tumor Registry. Gynecol Oncol 2017;147(3):521–7.

119. Conlon N, Schultheis AM, Piscuoglio S, et al. A survey of DICER1 hotspot mutations in ovarian and testicular sex cord-stromal tumors. Mod Pathol 2015;28(12):1603–12.

120. Kato N, Kusumi T, Kamataki A, et al. DICER1 hotspot mutations in ovarian Sertoli-Leydig cell tumors: a potential association with androgenic effects. Hum Pathol 2017;59:41–7.

121. Witkowski L, Mattina J, Schonberger S, et al. DICER1 hotspot mutations in nonepithelial gonadal tumours. Br J Cancer 2013;109(10):2744–50.

122. Karnezis AN, Wang Y, Keul J, et al. DICER1 and FOXL2 mutation status correlates with clinicopathologic features in ovarian Sertoli Leydig cell tumors. Am J Surg Pathol 2019;43(5):628–38.

123. Meyer R. Tubuläre (testiculäre) und solide Formen des Andreiblastoma ovarii und ihre Beziehung zur Vermännlichung. Beith Path Anat 1930;84:485–520.

124. Novak ER. Gynandroblastoma of the ovary: review of 8 cases from the ovarian tumor registry. Obstet Gynecol 1967;30(5):709–15.
125. Chivukula M, Hunt J, Carter G, et al. Recurrent gynandroblastoma of ovary-A case report: a molecular and immunohistochemical analysis. Int J Gynecol Pathol 2007;26(1):30–3.
126. Mercier AM, Zorn KK, Quick CM, et al. Recurrent gynandroblastoma of the ovary with germline DICER1 mutation: a case report and review of the literature. Gynecol Oncol Rep 2021;37:100806.
127. Wang Y, Karnezis AN, Magrill J, et al. DICER1 hot-spot mutations in ovarian gynandroblastoma. Histopathology 2018;73(2):306–13.
128. Oparka R, Cassidy A, Reilly S, et al. The C134W (402 C>G) FOXL2 mutation is absent in ovarian gynandroblastoma: insights into the genesis of an unusual tumour. Histopathology 2012;60(5):838–42.
129. Ordulu Z, Young RH. Sertoli-Leydig cell tumors of the ovary with follicular differentiation often resembling juvenile granulosa cell tumor: a report of 38 cases including comments on sex cord-stromal tumors of mixed forms (So-called Gynandroblastoma). Am J Surg Pathol 2021;45(1):59–67.
130. Jarzembowski JA, Lieberman RW. Pediatric sex cord-stromal tumor with composite morphology: a case report. Pediatr Dev Pathol 2005;8(6):680–4.
131. Young RH, Scully RE. Ovarian stromal tumors with minor sex cord elements: a report of seven cases. Int J Gynecol Pathol 1983;2(3):227–34.
132. Boyraz B, Watkins JC, Soubeyran I, Bonhomme B, Croce S, Oliva E, Young RH. Cystic Granulosa Cell Tumors of the Ovary. Arch Pathol Lab Med. 2022 Mar 30. https://doi.org/10.5858/arpa.2021-0385-OA. Epub ahead of print. PMID: 35353158.

Kidney Tumors
New and Emerging Kidney Tumor Entities

Farshid Siadat, MD, FRCPC[a], Mehdi Mansoor, MD, FRCPC[a],
Ondrej Hes, MD, PhD[b,1], Kiril Trpkov, MD, FRCPC[a,*]

KEYWORDS

- Kidney • Renal cell carcinoma • Unclassified renal tumor
- Unclassified renal cell carcinoma • Novel entities • Pathology • WHO • GUPS

KEY POINTS

- Several novel and emerging renal entities have been recently characterized, owing to the rapid acquisition of new evidence and knowledge.
- This review summarizes the current state of the art on several new and emerging renal entities, including eosinophilic solid and cystic renal cell carcinoma, renal cell carcinoma with fibromyomatous stroma, anaplastic lymphoma kinase-rearranged renal cell carcinoma, low-grade oncocytic renal tumor, eosinophilic vacuolated tumor, thyroid-like follicular renal cell carcinoma, and biphasic hyalinizing psammomatous renal cell carcinoma.
- Pathologists played a key role in characterizing these new and emerging tumors; importantly the diagnosis of most of them rests primarily on recognizing their morphologic features with the aid of immunohistochemistry.
- We hope that this updated review will promote awareness of these entities, and will stimulate additional studies for their further characterization, resulting in more accurate diagnosis and improved patient prognostication and management.

EOSINOPHILIC SOLID AND CYSTIC RENAL CELL CARCINOMA
Introduction

Eosinophilic solid and cystic renal cell carcinoma (ESC RCC) is a recently characterized renal cell neoplasm demonstrating a unique set of clinical, microscopic, immunohistochemical, and molecular features.[1,2] Such tumors were likely designated previously as "unclassified RCC" or "unclassified renal neoplasm/RCC with oncocytic/eosinophilic features."

This article originally appeared in *Surgical Pathology Clinics* Volume 15 Issue 4, December 2022.
[a] Department of Pathology and Laboratory Medicine, Cumming School of Medicine, University of Calgary, Rockyview General Hospital, 7007 14 Street, Calgary, Alberta T2V 1P9, Canada;
[b] Department of Pathology, Charles University in Prague, Faculty of Medicine in Plzeň, University Hospital Plzen, Alej Svobody 80, 304 60 Pilsen, Czech Republic
[1] Deceased July 2, 2022
* Corresponding author.
E-mail address: kiril.trpkov@albertaprecisionlabs.ca
Twitter: @FSiadat (F.S.); @Kiril_T_Can (K.T.)

Clinical Features

ESC RCC is typically sporadic and solitary tumor, found in patients of broad age range; most tumors are identified in females.[1-3] A subset has been documented in patients with tuberous sclerosis complex (TSC).[4,5] Although a great majority of ESC RCCs have indolent behavior, rare tumors with metastatic disease have also been reported, warranting the designation of "carcinoma" for this entity.[6-8]

Gross

As the descriptive name implies, solid and cystic components are the main gross features of ESC RCC. The tumors are well delineated, but nonencapsulated, and show a variable mix of solid parts and macrocysts. The cysts range from few millimeters to few centimeters. Rare cases have predominantly solid growth, with only rare microcysts. Tumor cut section is yellow, gray, and tan. Reported size varied broadly, but most tumors are less than 5 cm in size.[1,2]

Microscopy

The solid parts are composed of eosinophilic cells exhibiting diffuse, compact acinar, or nested growth (**Fig. 1**A–B).[1,2] Scattered foamy histiocytes and lymphocytes are also common, as are psammoma bodies. A characteristic feature is the presence of coarse, basophilic to purple, cytoplasmic granules (stippling). The nuclei are round to oval with focally prominent nucleoli. Focal papillary growth, clear cell areas, focal insular or tubular growth, and clusters of multinucleated cells can also be found.

Immunohistochemistry

ESC RCC shows either diffuse or focal CK20 expression (see **Fig. 1**C), although rare cases may be CK20 negative.[1,2] CK7 is typically negative or very focally positive. At least focal cathepsin K expression has been documented in a great majority of cases. Other positive stains include PAX8, AE1/AE3, CK8/18, and vimentin. Negative stains include CD117 and CAIX; HMB45 and melan-A are also negative in a great majority of cases, although rare cases show focal reactivity.

Molecular and Genetic Findings

Most sporadic ESC RCCs have recurrent, somatic biallelic losses or mutations in *TSC2* and *TSC1*. A subset of tumors has been identified in patients with TSC. These genetic changes result in dysregulation of the mammalian target of rapamycin (mTOR) signaling pathway.[6,9,10]

Differential Diagnosis

1. Oncocytoma: Typically lacks large cysts; cells have homogeneous oncocytic cytoplasm, without coarse granules. Immunohistochemistry (IHC): CD117+/CK20−/vimentin− (vs ESC RCC: CD117−/CK20+/vimentin+).
2. Chromophobe RCC, eosinophilic: Typically lacks large cysts, and cells lack coarse granules; irregular (raisinoid) nuclei with perinuclear halos are typical. IHC: CD117+/CK7+/CK20−/vimentin− (vs ESC RCC: CD117−/CK7−/CK20+/vimentin+).
3. SDH-deficient RCC: Cells have more flocculent cytoplasm and intracytoplasmic vacuoles. IHC: SDHB−/CK20−.
4. Epithelioid angiomyolipoma: Typically lacks large cysts (although smaller cysts can be present in some cases); cells lack coarse granules. IHC: PAX8−/CK20− (vs ESC RCC: PAX8+/CK20+).

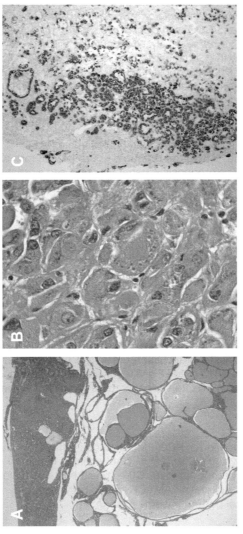

Fig. 1. ESC RCC. (*A*) At low power, it is an eosinophilic tumor that shows solid and cystic components; the cysts vary in size from macroscopic to microscopic. (*B*) The cells have voluminous eosinophilic cytoplasm with characteristic coarse cytoplasmic granules (stippling). (*C*) ESC RCC is typically CK20 positive (either diffuse or focal).

RENAL CELL CARCINOMA WITH FIBROMYOMATOUS STROMA
Introduction

Renal cell carcinoma with fibromyomatous stroma (RCC FMS) was described by Canzonieri and colleagues[11] in 1993, named as *mixed renal tumor with carcinomatous and fibroleiomyomatous components*. Over the years, various names were used in the literature to describe this entity, including: *RCC with prominent smooth muscle stroma, mixed renal tumor with carcinomatous and fibroleiomyomatous components, RCC associated with prominent angioleiomyoma-like proliferation, clear cell RCC with smooth muscle stroma*, and *RCC with clear cells, smooth muscle stroma, and negativity for 3p deletion*.[12] The name renal cell carcinoma with fibromyomatous stroma was officially endorsed by the Genitourinary Pathology Society (GUPS) in 2021, based on a broad consensus.[14] Recently published fifth edition of World Health Organization (WHO) classification of genitourinary tumors refers to this tumor as "renal cell carcinoma with prominent leiomyomatous stroma."[13]

Clinical Features

RCC FMS occurs more frequently in women (male:female [M:F] = 1:2) and is seen in adults of broad age range. The tumor is usually sporadic, but rare cases had familial association with TSC.[15] The prognosis is generally good and a great majority of cases had an indolent clinical course.[14,16,17] One case has been reported with lymph node metastasis in a patient with tuberous sclerosis and multifocal tumors.[18]

Gross

RCC FMS is a well-circumscribed, solid tumor, usually of small size (mean: 2.7 cm). Cut surface has a tan-brown color, often with lobulated appearance due to fibromyomatous septae.[12,19,20]

Microscopy

RCC FMS is typically composed of an epithelial neoplastic component, often forming nodules, separated by and admixed with a fibromuscular stromal component (**Fig. 2A**). The epithelial component consists of cells with voluminous clear cytoplasm, arranged in solid sheets, nests, branching tubules, and focal papillary structures (see **Fig. 2B–C**). The nuclei are WHO grade 2 or 3 (equivalent). The fibromyomatous stromal component can be variable and often appears more prominent at the periphery of the tumor.[12,14,19]

Immunohistochemistry

The characteristic IHC profile for RCC FMS includes diffuse positivity for CK7 (see **Fig. 2D**), as well as CAIX and CD10.[14,16,21] CAIX staining is usually diffuse membranous, but focally it can be cup shaped. Other positive stains include vimentin and high-molecular-weight cytokeratin. AMACR is typically negative. CK20 has been found positive in an apical pattern in some cases.[22]

Molecular and Genetic Findings

Molecular studies have provided evidence of association of RCC FMS with mutations involving the TSC/MTOR pathway.[14,16,22] A subset of tumors has shown mutations of *ELOC* (previously known as *TCEB1*) and monosomy of chromosome 8.[23] Unlike conventional clear cell RCC, these tumors are not associated with loss of heterozygosity (LOH) in chromosome 3p or *VHL* mutations.[14,24] Fibromyomatous stroma has been shown to be polyclonal and nonneoplastic.[24]

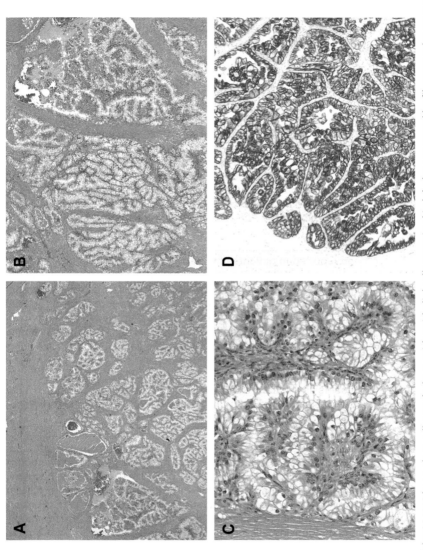

Fig. 2. RCC FMS. (*A*) RCC FMS has a clear cell morphology, with epithelial cells organized in lobules, separated by fibromuscular stroma. (*B*) The epithelial component often forms compact branching tubules (left) and focal papillary formations (*right*). (*C*) At high power, the nuclei are enlarged and may show more prominent nucleoli. (*D*) CK7 is typically diffusely positive.

Differential Diagnosis

1. Clear cell RCC: Typically lacks fibromyomatous stroma (although rare cases may show focally prominent stroma). Focal papillary structures are not usually present. IHC: CK7 is negative (or only focally positive); CD10 and AMACR are usually positive.
2. Clear cell papillary renal cell tumor: Cells have scant clear cytoplasm and form tubular and focal papillary structures. The nuclei are of lower grade (WHO/ISUP grade1 equivalent) and have a linear arrangement along the luminal surface. IHC: diffuse positivity for CAIX (cup shaped, not box shaped) and CK7, but CD10 is negative, as is AMACR.

ANAPLASTIC LYMPHOMA KINASE-REARRANGED RENAL CELL CARCINOMA
Introduction

Anaplastic lymphoma kinase-rearranged renal cell carcinoma (ALK RCC) is a renal entity first described in 2011.[25,26] ALK RCC is listed in the 2022 fifth edition of WHO classification of genitourinary tumors as a molecularly defined entity.[13] ALK RCC is characterized by an *ALK* gene fusion with various partner genes, leading to aberrant *ALK* activation. *ALK* rearrangement can be identified either by ALK protein expression on IHC, fluorescence in situ hybridization (FISH), or by sequencing methods. ALK RCC is a clinically important diagnosis because targeted therapies with ALK inhibitors are available and can be used as in other *ALK* rearrangement-associated neoplasms.[27,28]

Clinical Features

ALK RCCs have been reported in patients of wide age range, including pediatric and adolescent patients with sickle cell trait, as well as adult patients who typically did not harbor a sickle cell trait.[29] ALK RCC is not associated with other extrarenal tumors harboring ALK rearrangement. ALK RCC is slightly more common in males (M:F = 1.5:1). Patients had a diverse racial background, including African American, Caucasian, and Asian. ALK RCCs are indolent in most cases, although some may show aggressive clinical course, including metastasis and death.

Gross

ALK RCC usually presents as a solitary and circumscribed tumor, often less than 5 cm in size; it may be solid or solid-cystic, with tan-gray or variegated cut surface. Pseudocapsule of varying thickness can also be found.

Microscopy

ALK RCC typically demonstrates variable and diverse morphology with no characteristic or specific morphologic features. The growth patterns may include papillary, solid, tubular, trabecular cystic, cribriform, signet-ring, single cells, "mucinous tubular and spindle cell RCC-like" and "metanephric adenoma-like" (**Fig. 3**A–C).[14,29] However, mucinous or myxoid component (intracellular or interstitial) has been commonly found. Thus, a diagnostic consideration of ALK RCC and screening for ALK should be done in all difficult-to-classify renal tumors with variable and admixed patterns, unusual morphologies, or containing a mucinous component. Psammoma bodies and tumor necrosis are also common.

Immunohistochemistry

ALK protein expression by IHC, typically diffuse cytoplasmic and membranous, is a defining feature of ALK RCC (see **Fig. 3**D). Remaining immunoprofile is nonspecific

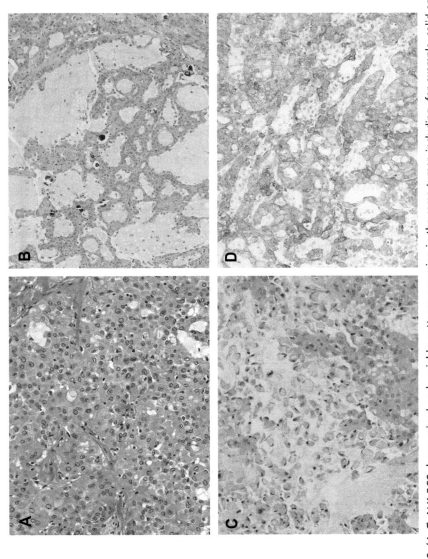

Fig. 3. ALK RCC. (A–C) ALK RCC shows mixed and variable patterns occurring in the same tumor, including, for example, solid areas (A); papillary, trabecular and tubulocystic areas, often with scattered psammomatous calcification (B); and focal single signet-ring cells (C). Note the extracellular mucinous background (B) and intracellular mucin in the signet-ring cells (C). (D) ALK expression is uniformly positive.

and includes reactivity for PAX8, CK7, vimentin, INI1 (retained), 34βE12, and AMACR. Negative IHC stains include CK20, GATA3, melan-A, HMB45, S100, and cathepsin K.[14,29] TFE3 reactivity by IHC was reported in some cases, but without evidence of *TFE3* rearrangement by FISH.[30]

Molecular and Genetic Findings

Several *ALK* fusion partners were identified in ALK RCC, including *VCL, HOOK1, STRN, TPM3, EML4,* and *PLEKHA7.*[14] A recent multi-institutional study reported 3 additional fusion partners *CLIP1, KIF5B,* and *KIAA1217.*[29]

Differential Diagnosis

The differential diagnosis of ALK RCC is broad, because its heterogeneous morphology may mimic a wide spectrum of other renal tumors, including SMARCB1-deficient renal medullary carcinoma (in children and adolescents), papillary RCC, MiTF RCC (TFE3 and TFEB), rhabdoid RCC (or clear cell RCC with rhabdoid features), collecting duct carcinoma, metanephric adenoma, mucinous tubular and spindle cell RCC, or unclassifiable RCC/tumor. A negative ALK IHC along with more specific immunomarkers for certain entities may help rule out ALK RCC.

EOSINOPHILIC VACUOLATED TUMOR
Introduction

Eosinophilic vacuolated tumor (EVT) is a recently described renal entity that emerged from the group of eosinophilic/oncocytic tumors with shared features between renal oncocytoma and chromophobe RCC.[31–33] EVT was described by He and colleagues[34] (as high-grade oncocytic tumor [HOT])[34] and by Chen and colleagues[35] (as sporadic RCC with eosinophilic and vacuolated cytoplasm). The recent GUPS consensus proposed the name *eosinophilic vacuolated tumor* for this entity.[14] EVT was also identified in some patients with TSC.[22,36–38] The 2022 fifth edition of WHO classification regards this tumor as one of the two emerging entities within the broader category of "other oncocytic tumors."[13]

Clinical Features

EVT is found in patients of broad age range and occurs more frequently in women (M:F = 1:2.5).[14,34,35,39] All reported EVT cases had benign behavior, without evidence of recurrence or metastatic disease.[14,39,40]

Gross

EVT is mostly a solitary and sporadic tumor of smaller size, about 3 to 4 cm in greatest dimension, although rare EVTs have been documented exceeding 10 cm.[34,35,38,39] EVT is typically solid, gray, or tan to brown tumor.[14,34,35,38,39]

Microscopy

EVT has a diffuse and solid growth, often admixed with nested and tubulocystic foci. Thick-walled vessels are virtually always present at the periphery, but a well-formed capsule is lacking. The cells have an eosinophilic cytoplasm and prominent intracytoplasmic vacuoles (**Fig. 4**A). The nuclei are round to oval, with prominent nucleoli that focally can be quite large and resemble viral inclusion.[34,35]

Immunohistochemistry and Electron Microscopy

EVT is positive for CD117 (KIT), CD10, antimitochondrial antigen antibody, and cathepsin K, in some cases focally (see **Fig. 4**B); CK7 is typically expressed only in

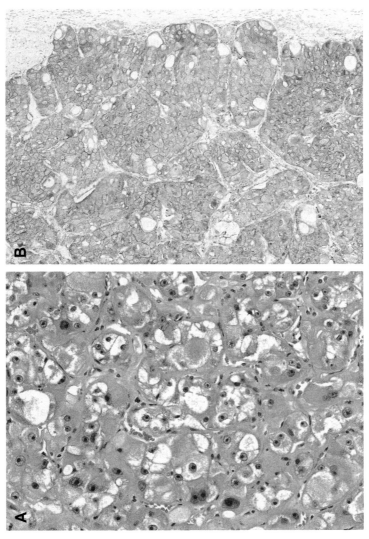

Fig. 4. EVT. (A) EVT is composed of eosinophilic cells with voluminous cytoplasm, typically showing prominent intracytoplasmic vacuoles, and enlarged, round to oval nuclei, often with very prominent nucleoli, imparting a "high-grade" appearance. (B) Cathepsin K is typically positive.

rare, scattered cells.[34,39] The immunoprofile "CD117+ and CK7+ only in rare cells" resembles that of an oncocytoma. EVT is negative for vimentin. Fumarate hydratase (FH) and succinate dehydrogenase B (SDHB) are retained. p-S6 and p-4EBP1, markers associated with mTOR pathway activation, have also been found to be expressed in EVT.[35]

On electron microscopy, EVT demonstrated numerous intracytoplasmic mitochondria, as well as dilated cisterns of rough endoplasmic reticulum.[38,40]

Molecular and Genetic Findings

Losses of chromosomes 1 and 19p were frequently found in EVT, along with loss of heterozygosity at 16p11 and 7q31.[34] However, complete losses or gains of other chromosomes, as in chromophobe RCC, have not been found. TSC/mTOR mutations seem to be consistent molecular findings in EVT[35,38] In a recent study, Farcas and colleagues[39] demonstrated nonoverlapping mutations in MTOR, TSC2, and TSC1 in all evaluated cases, associated with low mutational burden. Thus, EVT is associated with either germline or somatic mutations leading to mTORC1 activation.[38]

Differential Diagnosis

1. Hybrid oncocytic tumor (Birt-Hogg Dubé syndrome): Typically multiple/bilateral tumors with hybrid (oncocytoma/chromophobe RCC-like) look; no stromal areas; often scattered cells with clear cytoplasm (mosaic pattern); the nuclei are typically low-grade and without prominent nucleoli; may show perinuclear halos. IHC: CD117+, CK7+ only focally, cathepsin K+/− (limited data).
2. Oncocytoma: Can show tubulocystic growth; cells lack perinuclear halos; stromal archipelaginous areas are present containing larger cell aggregates. IHC: CD117+, CK7+ only in scattered cells, but cathepsin K− and often CD10−.
3. Chromophobe RCC, classic: Cells usually have more prominent membranes and show irregular (raisinoid) nuclei with uniform perinuclear halos. IHC: CD117+, CK7+, but cathepsin K− and often CD10−.
4. SDH-deficient RCC: Cells have more flocculent cytoplasm and intracytoplasmic vacuoles; lack perinuclear halos. Edematous stromal areas with individual cells (as in LOT) can be seen. IHC: SDHB−/CD117−/CK7−.

LOW-GRADE ONCOCYTIC TUMOR
Introduction

Low-grade oncocytic tumor (LOT) is another recently described renal tumor that emerged from the spectrum of eosinophilic/oncocytic tumors with shared features between renal oncocytoma and chromophobe RCC.[12,41] Rare examples have been found in patients with TSC.[42] LOT is another emerging entity included within the broader category of "other oncocytic tumors" in the fifth edition of the 2022 WHO classification.[13]

Clinical Features

LOT is typically found as a single and incidental tumor, but multiple LOTs have also been documented, either in patients with end-stage kidney disease[43] or in patients with TSC.[42] Lerma and colleagues[37] recently reported four patients, in whom LOT was associated with other recently described renal tumors, typically found in patients with TSC, including eosinophilic solid and cystic ESC RCC, EVT, RCC FMS, as well as angiomyolipoma and papillary adenoma.[37]

LOT was identified in patients of broad age range, but usually older patients. Overall, LOT is slightly more frequent in females (M:F = 1:1.3). All reported LOTs with available follow-up have behaved in a benign fashion, without evidence of disease progression and metastatic disease.[41–46]

Gross

LOT is usually a smaller tumor with median size between 3 and 4 cm, but similar to EVT; larger tumors have also been reported, exceeding 10 cm.[41,43,44] Grossly, LOT is a solid and compact tumor, without necrosis or cysts. Cut surface is tan-yellow to mahogany-brown, similar to oncocytoma.[41] Hemorrhagic areas may also be seen, usually more centrally.

Microscopy

LOT has a diffuse and solid growth, typically showing compact nests, and focal tubular, tubuloreticular, or trabecular growth. LOT lacks a well-formed capsule, and entrapped tubules may be seen at the periphery.[14,41] The neoplastic cells are eosinophilic with round to oval nuclei, lacking significant irregularities, and may show focal perinuclear halos or clearings (**Fig. 5A–B**). An important finding is that of sharply delineated, edematous stromal areas with scattered individual cells that can be elongated, and may form cordlike formations ("boats in a bay"), or may have an irregular "tissue culture" arrangement.[14,41] Edematous areas often contain fresh hemorrhage. Small lymphocytic collections can also be often seen in the solid areas.[14,41] Adverse features, such as coagulative necrosis, nuclear pleomorphism, cell atypia, multinucleation, and mitotic activity are typically absent.

Immunohistochemistry and Electron Microscopy

LOT is diffusely positive for CK7 (see **Fig. 5C**) and is negative, or in rare cases, very focally and weakly positive for CD117. LOT is also positive for PAX8, e-cadherin, BerEP4, and MOC31.[41] Negative stains include CAIX, CK20, CK5/6, p63, CD15, HMB45, melan-A, cathepsin K, and vimentin. CD10 and AMACR can be either negative or focally positive. FH and SDHB are retained. LOT is consistently positive for GATA3. LOT also expresses, at least focally, p-S6 and p-4EBP1, both markers associated with mTOR pathway activation.[42,45] Another novel marker FOXI1, typically expressed in both oncocytoma and chromophobe RCC, has been recently found to be negative or with very low reactivity in LOT.[47,48] In the normal kidney, FOXI1 is positive in the intercalated cells.[48]

On electron microscopy, LOT exhibits abundant, closely packed cytoplasmic mitochondria, similar to oncocytoma.[40]

Molecular and Genetic Features

LOT shows frequent deletions at 19p13, 1p36, and 19q13, or may show a disomic chromosomal status.[41] No other complete chromosomal gains or losses were found. CCND1 rearrangements are not found in LOT (unlike in oncocytoma, in which they are frequent).[43]

Recent studies demonstrated common involvement of the mTOR pathway genes in LOT. In one study, abnormalities in mTOR pathway genes were found in 80% (8 of 10) of evaluated LOTs, including mTOR (7 of 8) and TSC1 (1 of 8).[45] Another study found somatic, likely activating, mutations in mTOR (4 of 6) and RHEB (1 of 6) in 6 evaluable LOTs; one additional patient with multiple bilateral LOTs had a pathogenic germline mutation in TSC1 (1 of 6).[42] TSC1 germline mutations were also found in 2 patients with TSC mutations who had multiple LOTs.[37]

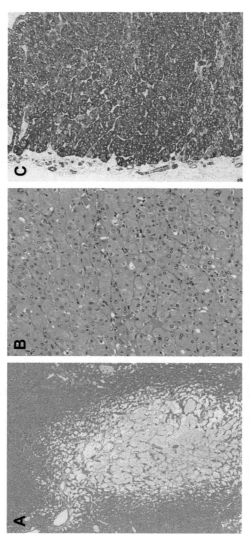

Fig. 5. LOT. (A) At low power, LOT is an eosinophilic solid tumor, often exhibiting sharply delineated, edematous areas with scattered individual cells ("boats in a bay"). (B). Higher magnification reveals eosinophilic cells with "low-grade" round to oval nuclei, and occasional perinuclear clearings. (C) EVT is diffusely positive for CK7 (shown) and negative for CD117 (not shown).

Differential Diagnosis

1. Oncocytoma: Can show tubulocystic growth, cells lack perinuclear halos, and archipelaginous areas are present containing larger cell aggregates. IHC: CD117+, CK7+ only in scattered cells.
2. Chromophobe RCC, eosinophilic: Lacks hypocellular stromal areas, cells usually have irregular (raisinoid) nuclei with uniform perinuclear halos. IHC: CD117+, CK7+.
3. SDH-deficient RCC: Cells have more flocculent cytoplasm and intracytoplasmic vacuoles, lack perinuclear halos. Edematous stromal areas with individual cells (as in LOT) may be present. IHC: SDHB−, CD117−, CK7−.

THYROID-LIKE FOLLICULAR RENAL CELL CARCINOMA
Introduction

Thyroid-like follicular renal cell carcinoma (TLF RCC) is a rare tumor with less than 50 cases described in the literature, mostly published as individual case reports. TLF RCC has also been considered an emerging renal entity in the recent GUPS update[14] and is listed in the 2022 fifth edition of WHO as an "emerging entity."[13]

Clinical Features

The sex distribution of TLF RCC has a slight female predominance (M:F = 1:1.8). Age range is broad (from 10 to 83 years).[49–51] No specific clinical features have been associated with TLF RCC. The clinical behavior was usually indolent in most reported cases, but lymph node and distant metastases were documented in about 10% of the patients.[52–55] Some reports have documented associations in individual patients with a family history of hereditary leiomyomatosis-associated RCC but without *FH* mutation, with mixed epithelial stromal tumor of the kidney, nephrolithiasis, and polycystic kidney disease.[14,54,56–59]

Gross

TLF RCC is a solitary, solid, well-circumscribed, and nonencapsulated tumor. The reported size range was wide (from 0.8 to 16.5 cm).[14,49–51]

Microscopy

TLF RCC resembles thyroid gland morphology (**Fig. 6A–B**). The tumors demonstrated follicular pattern, but focal branching and papillary structures were also reported. The size of the follicles was variable, and they were typically lined by a single layer of cuboidal or low columnar epithelial cells. The reported WHO grade was 2 or 3 (equivalent).[12,14,49–52,60–63] Sarcomatoid differentiation has been reported in one case.[64]

Immunohistochemistry

TLF RCC is usually positive for CK7, vimentin, and PAX8, and less frequently for RCC, AMACR, CD10, and CK20. An important finding is the negative staining for TTF1 and thyroglobulin, in contrast to true metastatic carcinomas of the thyroid.[14,58]

Molecular and Genetic Features

An association of TLF RCC and *EWSR1* gene abnormality has been recently reported by Al-Obaidy and colleagues,[58] documenting a fusion of *EWSR1-PATZ1* genes in 3 cases. The reported copy number variations have been variable, but neither consistent copy number changes nor other recurrent gene alterations have been found in TLF RCC.[49,55,60,64–66]

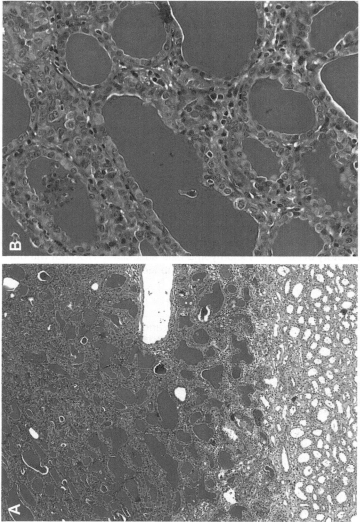

Fig. 6. TLF RCC. (*A*) This tumor shows a morphology resembling a thyroid gland, and is composed of back-to-back arranged, variable-sized follicles, with "colloid-like" luminal content. (*B*) At high power, the follicles are lined by a single layer of cuboidal to low columnar epithelial cells.

Differential Diagnosis

1. Metastasis of thyroid gland carcinoma to the kidney: This is the most important differential diagnosis that can be easily ruled out by IHC, because TTF1+ and thyroglobulin+ are found in a thyroid metastasis, in contrast to TLF RCC, which is negative for both. Caution: metastatic thyroid carcinoma is PAX8+, which may be a pitfall, because PAX8+ is found in almost all thyroid gland tumors.
2. Atrophic kidney-like lesion: Rare, well-demarcated, brown, tumor-like mass; considered nonneoplastic and likely reactive. This lesion is composed of atrophic renal tubules admixed with rare collapsed glomeruli. The key morphologic findings are the atrophic tubules and the collapsed glomeruli, which are not found in TLF RCC.

BIPHASIC HYALINIZING PSAMMOMATOUS RENAL CELL CARCINOMA
Introduction

Biphasic hyalinizing psammomatous renal cell carcinoma (BHP RCC) is a recently proposed renal tumor entity, invariably demonstrating neurofibromin 2 *(NF2)* mutations.[67] However, it is unclear whether *NF2* abnormalities represent a specific feature or a genetic driver in a group of related tumors that may represent an entity, or if they are a nonspecific finding, because they have been found in other RCC subtypes with various morphologies.[67–69] For example, in one recent study, 2 tumors described as BHP RCC did not show *NF2* abnormality.[70] In contrast, *NF2* abnormalities have been identified in some advanced papillary RCCs.[69] Thus, further study is necessary to validate whether BHP RCC represents a distinct renal entity sharing *NF2* gene abnormalities.[14,68,71]

Clinical Features

No specific clinical features were identified in the initial series of 8 cases,[67] and in a subsequent series of 6 cases.[72] There were 6 males and 1 female (1 unknown gender) in the study by Argani and colleagues,[67] and 3 males and 3 females in the study by Wang and colleagues.[72] Age range was broad (39–82 years), and no hereditary/syndromic or other associations were reported. Approximately half of the cases reported in the literature demonstrated metastatic disease.[70,71]

Gross

BHP RCC is a well-demarcated, solid, solitary tumor, occasionally demonstrating a peripheral capsule. Size ranged from 0.9 to 7.5 cm.[67,70–73]

Microscopy

BHP RCC is a solid tumor, with variable architecture, often including papillary and tubular growth. The tumors were typically composed of biphasic neoplastic cells, with smaller cells clustering around basement membrane material forming pseudorosettes and resembling the classic morphology of TFEB RCC (**Fig. 7**A–B). The second cell population consisted of larger cells with pale cytoplasm. Some reported tumors resembled a gonadoblastoma and formed solid pseudotubules or pseudoresettes, composed of cuboidal to cylindrical cells with pale to eosinophilic cytoplasm. Another morphologic variation was the presence of focal tubulopapillary growth, associated with basement membrane material, resulting in a glomeruloid appearance. The stromal component was typically sclerotic and focally hyalinized and scattered psammoma bodies were common.[67,71–73]

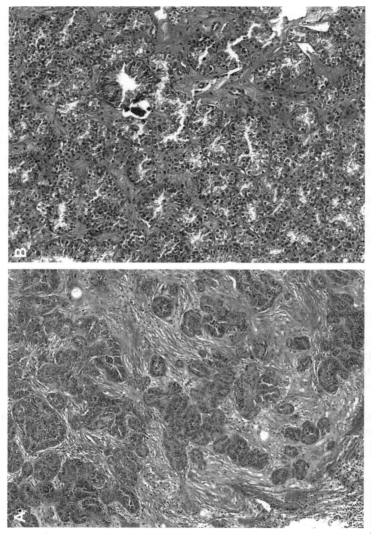

Fig. 7. BHP RCC. (*A*) BHP RCC is a solid tumor composed of glandlike structures, embedded in a fibrous, focally hyalinized stroma. These tumors typically show biphasic cell composition with smaller cells forming pseudorosettes. (*B*) Some areas show tubular morphology, and scattered psammoma bodies are common.

Table 1
Features of novel and emerging renal entities

Type	Clinical Features	Morphology	Immunohistochemistry	Molecular Features
ESC RCC	Mostly in females, mostly sporadic and solitary, rare cases in patients with TSC, indolent (great majority)	Solid and cystic, voluminous eosinophilic cells, cytoplasmic stippling	CK20+ CK7– CD117–v imentin+c athepsin K+ (focal)	Somatic biallelic loss or mutations of TSC1 and TSC2
RCC FMS	Mostly sporadic and solitary, rare cases in patients with TSC, indolent (great majority)	Solid, smaller tumor, tan to brown, frequent lobulated appearance; clear cells with voluminous cytoplasm forming nodules, separated and encircled by fibromuscular stroma	CK7+ CAIX+ (membranous) CD10+ AMACR–	Frequent mutations in TSC/mTOR pathway genes, ELOC (TCEB1) mutation in some cases; some lack VHL mutations, or LOH/deletion of chromosome 3
ALK RCC	Broad age range, solitary tumor, some in patients with sickle cell trait	Diverse (variable admixed patterns), often mucinous/myxoid background; medullary carcinoma-like morphology in children	ALK+ Other IHC nonspecific Rare cases TFE3+ (without translocation)	ALK rearrangement Fusion partners: VCL, HOOK1, STRN, TPM3, EML4, PLEKHA7, CLIP1, KIF5B, and KIAA1217
EVT	Broad age range, sporadic and solitary, rare cases in patients with TSC, indolent	Solid, smaller tumor, tan to brown or gray, large vessels often found at the periphery; eosinophilic cells with frequent and prominent intracytoplasmic vacuoles, large nucleoli	cathepsin K+ CD117+ CD10+ CK7– (only rare cells +) CK20–v imentin–	TSC/mTOR mutations virtually in all cases, deletions of chromosome 19 and 1 also found

(continued on next page)

Table 1
(continued)

Type	Clinical Features	Morphology	Immunohistochemistry	Molecular Features
LOT	Older patients, sporadic and solitary, rare cases in patients with TSC, indolent	Solid, smaller tumor, tan to mahogany brown; sharp transition to edematous areas with scattered individual cells; round to oval nuclei without irregularities and prominent nucleoli, often with perinuclear halos	CK7+ (diffuse) CD117– (rarely weak +) GATA3+ (limited data) FOXI1– CK20–v imentin–	Frequent *TSC/MTOR* mutations, lacks multiple chromosomal losses, deletions of chromosomes 19p, 19q and 1p also found, no *CCND1* rearrangements
TLF RCC	Broad age range including children, solitary, mostly indolent	Thyroid-like follicular arrangement, follicles of variable size with eosinophilic luminal content, lining cells cuboidal to cylindrical	CK7+ PAX8+ Vimentin– TTF1–t hyroglobulin–	Fusion of *EWSR1-PATZ1* found in 3 cases No other specific findings
BHP RCC	Adult patients, about half of tumors with aggressive clinical course	Tubulopapillary architecture, prominent fibrotic to hyalinized stroma, and microcalcifications Heterogeneous morphology	CK7+ PAX8+ CD10+ HMB45–m elan A–	*NF2* abnormalities, loss of chromosome 22 found in some cases

Immunohistochemistry

The neoplastic cells were usually reactive for PAX8, CD10, and CK7, but were negative for GATA3, cathepsin K, melan-A, inhibin, SF1, and WT1. All tested cases were also negative for *TFE3* and *TFEB* rearrangements by break-apart FISH.

Molecular and Genetic Features

A typical molecular feature identified in all analyzable cases of BHP RCC was a mutations of the *NF2* gene.[67,71,72] In a recent study, two tumors described as BHP RCC lacked *NF2* abnormalities.[70] Additional mutations in *PBMRT1, BAP1, ARID1A, DNMT3A, TERT*, and *SMARCB1* were also found in some cases. The copy number variation pattern was not uniform and showed multiple chromosomal gains and losses, most commonly a loss of chromosome 22. Coalteration of *NF2* and *PBMRT1* was found in some cases with aggressive clinical course.[71]

Differential Diagnosis

BHP RCC represents a heterogeneous group of renal tumors with a limited number of reported cases, usually demonstrating prominent fibrotic and hyalinized stroma, microcalcification, and tubulopapillary architecture. The differential diagnosis of BHP RCC is broad and may include papillary RCC, MiTF family RCC (often demonstrating cathepsin K or melanotic marker expression, as well as *TFE3/TFEB* rearrangements), *ALK*-rearranged RCC (typically showing ALK rearrangements), and metastatic sex core stromal tumor, such as gonadoblastoma (which can be ruled out by the absence of gonadal primary and inhibin and SF1 immunoreactivity). However, without genetic testing for *NF2*, the diagnosis of BHP RCC remains virtually impossible.

SUMMARY

This article provides an overview of several new and emerging renal entities. The summary of their key features is shown in **Table 1**. The awareness of these renal neoplasms is essential for practicing pathologists because the navigation through this evolving field is a challenging task, even in places with large volumes of renal tumors. Such cases can, however, be seen in practices of any scope, and their correct classification requires diagnostic awareness among general pathologists, because they can be often diagnosed, or at least suspected, on morphology in combination with IHC. The recognition of such novel renal entities will guide both pathologists and clinicians in translating these developments into more accurate diagnosis and better patient management.

DISCLOSURE

Authors have no conflicts of interest to declare that are relevant to the content of this article.

DEDICATION

We dedicate this paper to our friend and colleague Dr. Ondřej Hes - Ondra, who passed away suddenly on July 2, 2022. We acknowledge and salute his many contributions that shaped the contemporary field of renal tumor pathology and resulted in recognition of many renal entities and subtypes included in this review and in the WHO 2022 classification (5th edition) of urinary and male genital tumors. We dedicate this paper to Dr. Hes to honor his memory, friendship, and scientific legacy.

REFERENCES

1. Trpkov K, Hes O, Bonert M, et al. Eosinophilic, Solid, and Cystic Renal Cell Carcinoma: Clinicopathologic Study of 16 Unique, Sporadic Neoplasms Occurring in Women. Am J Surg Pathol 2016;40(1):60–71.

2. Trpkov K, Abou-Ouf H, Hes O, et al. Eosinophilic Solid and Cystic Renal Cell Carcinoma (ESC RCC): Further Morphologic and Molecular Characterization of ESC RCC as a Distinct Entity. Am J Surg Pathol 2017;41(10):1299–308.

3. Li Y, Reuter VE, Matoso A, et al. Re-evaluation of 33 'unclassified' eosinophilic renal cell carcinomas in young patients. Histopathology 2018;72(4):588–600.

4. Guo J, Tretiakova MS, Troxell ML, et al. Tuberous Sclerosis-associated Renal Cell Carcinoma: A Clinicopathologic Study of 57 Separate Carcinomas in 18 Patients. Am J Surg Pathol 2014;38(11):1457–67.

5. Schreiner A, Daneshmand S, Bayne A, et al. Distinctive morphology of renal cell carcinomas in tuberous sclerosis. Int J Surg Pathol 2010;18(5):409–18.

6. Palsgrove DN, Li Y, Pratilas CA, et al. Eosinophilic Solid and Cystic (ESC) Renal Cell Carcinomas Harbor TSC Mutations: Molecular Analysis Supports an Expanding Clinicopathologic Spectrum. Am J Surg Pathol 2018;42(9):1166–81.

7. McKenney JK, Przybycin CG, Trpkov K, et al. Eosinophilic solid and cystic renal cell carcinomas have metastatic potential. Histopathology 2018;72(6):1066–7.

8. Tretiakova MS. Eosinophilic solid and cystic renal cell carcinoma mimicking epithelioid angiomyolipoma: series of 4 primary tumors and 2 metastases. Hum Pathol 2018;80:65–75.

9. Mehra R, Vats P, Cao X, et al. Somatic Bi-allelic Loss of TSC Genes in Eosinophilic Solid and Cystic Renal Cell Carcinoma. Eur Urol 2018;74(4):483–6.

10. Tjota M, Chen H, Parilla M, et al. Eosinophilic Renal Cell Tumors With a TSC and MTOR Gene Mutations Are Morphologically and Immunohistochemically Heterogenous: Clinicopathologic and Molecular Study. Am J Surg Pathol 2020;44(7):943–54.

11. Canzonieri V, Volpe R, Gloghini A, et al. Mixed renal tumor with carcinomatous and fibroleiomyomatous components, associated with angiomyolipoma in the same kidney. Pathol Res Pract 1993;189(8):951–6 [discussion: 957-959].

12. Trpkov K, Hes O. New and emerging renal entities: a perspective post-WHO 2016 classification. Histopathology 2019;74(1):31–59.

13. WHO Classification of Tumours. Edited by the WHO Classification of Tumours Editorial Board. Urinary and male genital tumours. 5th edition. WHO classification of tumours series, 8. Lyon (France): International Agency for Research on Cancer; 2022. https://publications.iarc.fr.

14. Trpkov K, Williamson SR, Gill AJ, et al. Novel, emerging and provisional renal entities: The Genitourinary Pathology Society (GUPS) update on renal neoplasia. Mod Pathol 2021;34(6):1167–84.

15. Gournay M, Dugay F, Belaud-Rotureau MA, et al. Renal cell carcinoma with leiomyomatous stroma in tuberous sclerosis complex: a distinct entity. Virchows Arch 2021;478(4):793–9.

16. Shah RB, Stohr BA, Tu ZJ, et al. Renal Cell Carcinoma With Leiomyomatous Stroma" Harbor Somatic Mutations of TSC1, TSC2, MTOR, and/or ELOC (TCEB1): Clinicopathologic and Molecular Characterization of 18 Sporadic Tumors Supports a Distinct Entity. Am J Surg Pathol 2020;44(5):571–81.

17. Williamson SR, Hornick JL, Eble JN, et al. Renal Cell Carcinoma with Angioleiomyoma-Like Stroma and Clear Cell Papillary Renal Cell Carcinoma:

Exploring SDHB Protein Immunohistochemistry and the Relationship to Tuberous Sclerosis Complex. Hum Pathol 2018;75:10–5.

18. Gupta S, Lohse CM, Rowsey R, et al. Renal Neoplasia in Polycystic Kidney Disease: An Assessment of Tuberous Sclerosis Complex-associated Renal Neoplasia and PKD1/TSC2 Contiguous Gene Deletion Syndrome. Eur Urol 2021;S0302-2838(21):02161–8. https://doi.org/10.1016/j.eururo.2021.11.013. Online ahead of print.

19. Martignoni G, Brunelli M, Segala D, et al. Renal cell carcinoma with smooth muscle stroma lacks chromosome 3p and VHL alterations. Mod Pathol 2014;27(5): 765–74.

20. Parilla M, Alikhan M, Al-Kawaaz M, et al. Genetic Underpinnings of Renal Cell Carcinoma With Leiomyomatous Stroma. Am J Surg Pathol 2019;43(8):1135–44.

21. Williamson SR, Cheng L, Eble JN, et al. Renal cell carcinoma with angioleiomyoma-like stroma: clinicopathological, immunohistochemical, and molecular features supporting classification as a distinct entity. Mod Pathol 2015; 28(2):279–94.

22. Gupta S, Jimenez RE, Herrera-Hernandez L, et al. Renal Neoplasia in Tuberous Sclerosis: A Study of 41 Patients. Mayo Clin Proc 2021;96(6):1470–89.

23. Hakimi AA, Tickoo SK, Jacobsen A, et al. TCEB1-mutated renal cell carcinoma: a distinct genomic and morphological subtype. Mod Pathol 2015;28(6):845–53.

24. Petersson F, Martinek P, Vanecek T, et al. Renal Cell Carcinoma With Leiomyomatous Stroma: A Group of Tumors With Indistinguishable Histopathologic Features, But 2 Distinct Genetic Profiles: Next-Generation Sequencing Analysis of 6 Cases Negative for Aberrations Related to the VHL gene. Appl Immunohistochem Mol Morphol 2018;26(3):192–7.

25. Marino-Enriquez A, Ou WB, Weldon CB, et al. ALK rearrangement in sickle cell trait-associated renal medullary carcinoma. Genes Chromosomes Cancer 2011;50(3):146–53.

26. Debelenko LV, Raimondi SC, Daw N, et al. Renal cell carcinoma with novel VCL-ALK fusion: new representative of ALK-associated tumor spectrum. Mod Pathol 2011;24(3):430–42.

27. Pal SK, Bergerot P, Dizman N, et al. Responses to Alectinib in ALK-rearranged Papillary Renal Cell Carcinoma. Eur Urol 2018;74(1):124–8.

28. Hallberg B, Palmer RH. Mechanistic insight into ALK receptor tyrosine kinase in human cancer biology. Nat Rev Cancer 2013;13(10):685–700.

29. Kuroda N, Trpkov K, Gao Y, et al. ALK rearranged renal cell carcinoma (ALK-RCC): a multi-institutional study of twelve cases with identification of novel partner genes CLIP1, KIF5B and KIAA1217. Mod Pathol 2020;33(12):2564–79.

30. Thorner PS, Shago M, Marrano P, et al. TFE3-positive renal cell carcinomas are not always Xp11 translocation carcinomas: Report of a case with a TPM3-ALK translocation. Pathol Res Pract 2016;212(10):937–42.

31. Trpkov K, Hes O, Williamson SR, et al. New developments in existing WHO entities and evolving molecular concepts: The Genitourinary Pathology Society (GUPS) update on renal neoplasia. Mod Pathol 2021;34(7):1392–424.

32. Williamson SR, Gadde R, Trpkov K, et al. Diagnostic criteria for oncocytic renal neoplasms: a survey of urologic pathologists. Hum Pathol 2017;63:149–56.

33. Hes O, Petersson F, Kuroda N, et al. Renal hybrid oncocytic/chromophobe tumors - a review. Histol Histopathol 2013;28(10):1257–64.

34. He H, Trpkov K, Martinek P, et al. High-grade oncocytic renal tumor": morphologic, immunohistochemical, and molecular genetic study of 14 cases. Virchows Arch 2018;473(6):725–38.

35. Chen YB, Mirsadraei L, Jayakumaran G, et al. Somatic Mutations of TSC2 or MTOR Characterize a Morphologically Distinct Subset of Sporadic Renal Cell Carcinoma With Eosinophilic and Vacuolated Cytoplasm. Am J Surg Pathol 2019;43(1):121–31.

36. Trpkov K, Bonert M, Gao Y, et al. High-grade oncocytic tumour (HOT) of kidney in a patient with tuberous sclerosis complex. Histopathology 2019;75(3):440–2.

37. Lerma LA, Schade GR, Tretiakova MS. Co-existence of ESC-RCC, EVT, and LOT as synchronous and metachronous tumors in six patients with multifocal neoplasia but without clinical features of tuberous sclerosis complex. Hum Pathol 2021;116:1–11.

38. Kapur P, Gao M, Zhong H, et al. Eosinophilic Vacuolated Tumor of the Kidney: A Review of Evolving Concepts in This Novel Subtype With Additional Insights From a Case With MTOR Mutation and Concomitant Chromosome 1 Loss. Adv Anat Pathol 2021;28(4):251–7.

39. Farcas M, Gatalica Z, Trpkov K, et al. Eosinophilic vacuolated tumor (EVT) of kidney demonstrates sporadic TSC/MTOR mutations: next-generation sequencing multi-institutional study of 19 cases. Mod Pathol 2021. https://doi.org/10.1038/s41379-021-00923-6.

40. Siadat F, Trpkov K. ESC, ALK, HOT and LOT: Three Letter Acronyms of Emerging Renal Entities Knocking on the Door of the WHO Classification. Cancers (Basel) 2020;12(1).

41. Trpkov K, Williamson SR, Gao Y, et al. Low-grade Oncocytic Tumor of Kidney (CD117 Negative, Cytokeratin 7 Positive): A Distinct Entity? Histopathology 2019;75(2):174–84.

42. Kapur P, Gao M, Zhong H, et al. Germline and sporadic mTOR pathway mutations in low-grade oncocytic tumor of the kidney. Mod Pathol 2021. https://doi.org/10.1038/s41379-021-00896-6.

43. Kravtsov O, Gupta S, Cheville JC, et al. Low-Grade Oncocytic Tumor of Kidney (CK7-Positive, CD117-Negative): Incidence in a Single Institutional Experience with Clinicopathological and Molecular Characteristics. Hum Pathol 2021; 114:9–18.

44. Akgul M, Al-Obaidy KI, Cheng L, et al. Low-grade oncocytic tumour expands the spectrum of renal oncocytic tumours and deserves separate classification: a review of 23 cases from a single tertiary institute. J Clin Pathol 2021. https://doi.org/10.1136/jclinpath-2021-207478. jclinpath-2021-207478.

45. Morini A, Drossart T, Timsit MO, et al. Low-grade oncocytic renal tumor (LOT): mutations in mTOR pathway genes and low expression of FOXI1. Mod Pathol 2021. https://doi.org/10.1038/s41379-021-00906-7.

46. Guo Q, Liu N, Wang F, et al. Characterization of a distinct low-grade oncocytic renal tumor (CD117-negative and cytokeratin 7-positive) based on a tertiary oncology center experience: the new evidence from China. Virchows Arch 2020;449–58.

47. Tong K, Hu Z. FOXI1 expression in chromophobe renal cell carcinoma and renal oncocytoma: a study of The Cancer Genome Atlas transcriptome-based outlier mining and immunohistochemistry. Virchows Arch 2021;478(4):647–58.

48. Skala SL, Wang X, Zhang Y, et al. Next-generation RNA Sequencing-based Biomarker Characterization of Chromophobe Renal Cell Carcinoma and Related Oncocytic Neoplasms. Eur Urol 2020;78(1):63–74.

49. Amin MB, Gupta R, Ondrej H, et al. Primary thyroid-like follicular carcinoma of the kidney: report of 6 cases of a histologically distinctive adult renal epithelial neoplasm. Am J Surg Pathol 2009;33(3):393–400.

50. Alessandrini L, Fassan M, Gardiman MP, et al. Thyroid-like follicular carcinoma of the kidney: report of two cases with detailed immunohistochemical profile and literature review. Virchows Arch 2012;461(3):345–50.
51. Chen F, Wang Y, Wu X, et al. Clinical characteristics and pathology of thyroid-like follicular carcinoma of the kidney: Report of 3 cases and a literature review. Mol Clin Oncol 2016;4(2):143–50.
52. Dhillon J, Tannir NM, Matin SF, et al. Thyroid-like follicular carcinoma of the kidney with metastases to the lungs and retroperitoneal lymph nodes. Hum Pathol 2011; 42(1):146–50.
53. Vicens RA, Balachandran A, Guo CC, et al. Multimodality imaging of thyroid-like follicular renal cell carcinoma with lung metastases, a new emerging tumor entity. Abdom Imaging 2014;39(2):388–93.
54. Rao V, Menon S, Bakshi G, et al. Thyroid-Like Follicular Carcinoma of the Kidney With Low-Grade Sarcomatoid Component: A Hitherto Undescribed Case. Int J Surg Pathol 2021;29(3):327–33.
55. Ko JJ, Grewal JK, Ng T, et al. Whole-genome and transcriptome profiling of a metastatic thyroid-like follicular renal cell carcinoma. Cold Spring Harb Mol Case Stud 2018;4(6):a003137.
56. Wu WW, Chu JT, Nael A, et al. Thyroid-like follicular carcinoma of the kidney in a young patient with history of pediatric acute lymphoblastic leukemia. Case Rep Pathol 2014;2014:313974.
57. Volavsek M, Strojan-Flezar M, Mikuz G. Thyroid-like follicular carcinoma of the kidney in a patient with nephrolithiasis and polycystic kidney disease: a case report. Diagn Pathol 2013;8:108.
58. Al-Obaidy KI, Bridge JA, Cheng L, et al. EWSR1-PATZ1 fusion renal cell carcinoma: a recurrent gene fusion characterizing thyroid-like follicular renal cell carcinoma. Mod Pathol 2021;34:1921–34.
59. Tretiakova MS, Kehr EL, Gore JL, et al. Thyroid-Like Follicular Renal Cell Carcinoma Arising Within Benign Mixed Epithelial and Stromal Tumor. Int J Surg Pathol 2020;28(1):80–6.
60. Ohe C, Kuroda N, Pan CC, et al. A unique renal cell carcinoma with features of papillary renal cell carcinoma and thyroid-like carcinoma: a morphological, immunohistochemical and genetic study. Histopathology 2010;57(3):494–7.
61. Dhillon J, Mohanty SK, Krishnamurthy S. Cytologic diagnosis of thyroid-like follicular carcinoma of the kidney: a case report. Diagn Cytopathol 2014;42(3):273–7.
62. Dong L, Huang J, Huang L, et al. Thyroid-Like Follicular Carcinoma of the Kidney in a Patient with Skull and Meningeal Metastasis: A Unique Case Report and Review of the Literature. Medicine (Baltimore) 2016;95(15):e3314.
63. de Jesus LE, Fulgencio C, Leve T, et al. Thyroid-like follicular carcinoma of the kidney presenting on a 10 year-old prepubertal girl. Int Braz J Urol 2019;45(4): 834–42.
64. Jenkins TM, Rosenbaum J, Zhang PJ, et al. Thyroid-Like Follicular Carcinoma of the Kidney With Extensive Sarcomatoid Differentiation: A Case Report and Review of the Literature. Int J Surg Pathol 2019;27(6):678–83.
65. Jung SJ, Chung JI, Park SH, et al. Thyroid follicular carcinoma-like tumor of kidney: a case report with morphologic, immunohistochemical, and genetic analysis. Am J Surg Pathol 2006;30(3):411–5.
66. Fanelli GN, Fassan M, Dal Moro F, et al. Thyroid-like follicular carcinoma of the kidney: The mutational profiling reveals a BRAF wild type status. Pathol Res Pract 2019;215(9):152532.

67. Argani P, Reuter VE, Eble JN, et al. Biphasic Hyalinizing Psammomatous Renal Cell Carcinoma (BHP RCC): A Distinctive Neoplasm Associated With Somatic NF2 Mutations. Am J Surg Pathol 2020;44(7):901–16.
68. Chen YB, Xu J, Skanderup AJ, et al. Molecular analysis of aggressive renal cell carcinoma with unclassified histology reveals distinct subsets. Nat Commun 2016;7:13131.
69. Yakirevich E, Pavlick DC, Perrino CM, et al. NF2 Tumor Suppressor Gene Inactivation in Advanced Papillary Renal Cell Carcinoma. Am J Surg Pathol 2021;45(5): 716–8.
70. Chumbalkar V, Wang P, Paner GP. Spectrum of biphasic renal cell carcinomas with hyalinized stroma and psammoma bodies associated and not associated with NF2 alteration. Hum Pathol 2021. https://doi.org/10.1016/j.humpath.2021. 12.001. S0046-8177(21)00199-4.
71. Paintal A, Tjota MY, Wang P, et al. NF2-mutated Renal Carcinomas Have Common Morphologic Features Which Overlap With Biphasic Hyalinizing Psammomatous Renal Cell Carcinoma: A Comprehensive Study of 14 Cases. Am J Surg Pathol 2022. https://doi.org/10.1097/PAS.0000000000001846.
72. Wang G, Amin MB, Grossmann P, et al. Renal cell tumor with sex-cord/gonadoblastoma-like features: analysis of 6 cases. Virchows Arch 2021. https://doi.org/10.1007/s00428-021-03235-x.
73. Gopinath A, Mubeen A, Jamal M, et al. Biphasic Hyalinizing Psammomatous Renal Cell Carcinoma: Another Provisional Entity Emerging From the Papillary Renal Cell Carcinoma Pandora's Box. Int J Surg Pathol 2021;29(7):783–7.

A New Landscape of Testing and Therapeutics in Metastatic Breast Cancer

Geetha Jagannathan, MBBS[1], Marissa J. White, MD[1],
Rena R. Xian, MD[1,2], Leisha A. Emens, MD, PhD[3],
Ashley Cimino-Mathews, MD[1,2,*]

KEYWORDS

- Biomarkers • Metastasis • Breast cancer • PD-L1 • Tumor mutation burden
- Companion diagnostic

KEY POINTS

- Biomarker testing on metastatic breast carcinoma enables selection of targeted therapies, and companion diagnostics are required assays coupled to an associated therapy.
- The National Comprehensive Cancer Network (NCCN) recommends biomarker assessment of hormone receptor status, HER2, and *BRCA1/2* on all metastatic breast carcinomas, and suggests second-line biomarker assessment of *PIK3CA* on metastatic hormone receptor positive, HER2 negative carcinomas.
- The NCCN recommends biomarker assessment of PD-L1 on metastatic triple negative carcinomas, with assessment of tumor mutation burden, mismatch repair protein status/microsatellite instability, and *NTRK* status in select circumstances.

OVERVIEW

Metastatic breast cancer remains an incurable disease, with significantly lower 5-year survival (28%) compared with localized cancer (99%) and cancers with nodal involvement (86%).[1] The therapeutic options for patients with metastatic breast cancer were historically limited; however, research has generated new and promising targeted therapies for patients with metastatic breast cancer. Targeted therapies typically

This article originally appeared in *Surgical Pathology Clinics* Volume 15 Issue 1, March 2022.
[1] Department of Pathology, The Johns Hopkins University School of Medicine, 401 N Broadway, Weinberg 2242, Baltimore, MD 21287, USA; [2] Department of Oncology, The Johns Hopkins University School of Medicine, 401 N Broadway, Weinberg 2242, Baltimore, MD 21287, USA; [3] Department of Oncology, UPMC Hillman Cancer Center/Magee Women's Hospital, 5117 Centre Avenue, Room 1.46e, Pittsburgh, PA 15213, USA
* Corresponding author. 401 N Broadway, Weinberg 2242, Baltimore, MD 21287.
E-mail address: acimino1@jhmi.edu

require unique biomarker testing to determine eligibility for treatment, many of which must be performed with one particular assay.

The National Comprehensive Cancer Network (NCCN) clinical practice guidelines recommend assessment of the following biomarkers in metastatic breast cancer: hormone receptors, human epidermal growth factor receptor-2 (HER2), programmed death-ligand 1 (PD-L1) (in triple negative), and germline *BRCA1* and *BRCA2* status, with the option to test for *PIK3CA* as a second line in estrogen receptor (ER)-positive, HER2-negative cancers, and in select circumstances to test for mismatch repair protein status and tumor mutational burden and/or *NTRK* (**Tables 1–3**).[2] Recommended testing methods include immunohistochemistry (IHC), chromogenic in situ hybridization (CISH), fluorescent in situ hybridization (FISH), targeted gene sequencing, and large-panel next-generation sequencing. Many of these biomarkers must be determined using an assay that is designated by the US Food and Drug Administration (FDA) as a companion diagnostic for its associated targeted therapeutic agent.[3–5] In this review, we cover the recommended biomarker assessment, testing methods, and companion diagnostics for metastatic breast cancer.

Summary Box 1: Recommended biomarker assessment in metastatic breast cancer

1. Hormone receptors: ER and PR (all newly metastatic)

2. HER2 (all newly metastatic)

3. PD-L1 by 22C3 in triple-negative metastatic breast carcinomas

4. MSI or dMMR[a]

5. TMB[a]

6. *BRCA1* and *BRCA2* (germline testing on all newly metastatic patients)

7. *PIK3CA* (as a second-line option in ER-positive, HER2-negative metastatic cancer)

8. *NTRK*[a]

dMMR, mismatch repair protein deficiency; MSI, microsatellite instability; PD-L1, programmed death-ligand 1; PR, progesterone receptor; TMB, tumor mutation burden.

[a]In select circumstances.

HORMONE RECEPTOR AND HUMAN EPIDERMAL GROWTH FACTOR RECEPTOR-2 TESTING
Clinical Relevance

ER, progesterone receptor (PR), and HER2 testing are the prototype of predictive and prognostic biomarker testing in breast cancer. Retesting ER, PR, and HER2 on metastatic breast cancers at first occurrence, each recurrence, and on different sites of disease are standard of care. Based on their expression, breast cancers fall into 3 distinct prognostic and predictive groups: (1) hormone receptor positive and HER2 negative, (2) HER2 positive with or without hormone receptor expression, and (3) triple negative for both hormone receptors and HER2. Most often, metastatic disease has the same hormone receptor and HER2 expression profile as the primary tumor. However, a small but significant subset of the metastatic disease shows discordance in expression of these markers, which can significantly impact treatment decisions. In addition, tumoral heterogeneity and divergent clonal evolution can result in the presence of different hormone receptor or HER2 status in different tumor sites or in regions within one tumor (**Fig. 1**).[6,7]

Table 1
Biomarker characteristics for estrogen receptor, progesterone receptor, and human epidermal growth factor receptor-2

Marker	Breast Cancer Subtype Tested	Test Method	Sample Type	Scoring	Companion Diagnostics[5]	Manufacturer	FDA-Approved Drugs
ER and PR	Any	IHC	FFPE	Score intensity and percentage of tumor cells labeling: <1%: Negative ≥1%: Positive 1%–10% ER expression: Low positive	Any FDA-approved antibody platform. No formally designated companion diagnostic		Aromatase inhibitors; tamoxifen; CDK4/6 inhibitors with aromatase inhibitors or fulvestrant
HER2	Any	IHC	FFPE	Score intensity, completeness of membranous labeling and percentage of tumor cells labeling[14]. Negative (score 0 or 1+) Equivocal (2+) Positive (3+)	InSite Her-2/neu KIT	Biogenex Laboratories, Inc	Trastuzumab
					Bond Oracle HER2 IHC System	Leica Biosystems	Trastuzumab
					HercepTest	Dako Denmark A/S	Trastuzumab; pertuzumab; T-DM1
					PATHWAY anti- Her2/ neu (4B5) Rabbit Monoclonal Primary Antibody	Ventana Medical Systems, Inc	Trastuzumab; T-DM1
		FISH		Score average HER2 copy number and ratio of HER2 to CEP17 in tumor cells[15]	INFORM HER2 Dual ISH DNA Probe Cocktail	Ventana Medical Systems, Inc	Trastuzumab; T-DM1
					INFORM HER-2/neu	Ventana Medical Systems, Inc	Trastuzumab
					HER2 FISH pharmDx Kit	Dako Denmark A/s	Trastuzumab; Pertuzumab; T-DM1
					VENTANA HER2 Dual ISH DNA Probe Cocktail	Ventana Medical Systems, Inc	Trastuzumab
					PathVysion HER-2 DNA Probe Kit	Abbott Molecular Inc	Trastuzumab

(continued on next page)

Table 1
(continued)

Marker	Breast Cancer Subtype Tested	Test Method	Sample Type	Scoring	Companion Diagnostics[5]	Manufacturer	FDA-Approved Drugs
		CISH		Score average HER2 copy number in tumor cells	SPOT-Light HER2 CISH Kit	Life Technologies Corporation	Trastuzumab
		NGS			HER2 CISH pharmDx Kit FoundationOne CDx	Dako Denmark A/S Foundation Medicine, Inc	Trastuzumab Trastuzumab; pertuzumab; T-DM1

Abbreviations: CEP17, chromosome enumeration probe 17; CISH, chromogenic in situ hybridization; FFPE, formalin-fixed paraffin-embedded; FISH, fluorescence in situ hybridization; IHC, immunohistochemistry; NGS, next-generation sequencing; T-DM1, ado-trastuzumab emtansine.

Table 2
Biomarker characteristics for immunotherapy: programmed death-ligand 1, tumor mutation burden, and microsatellite instability/mismatch repair protein deficiency

Marker	Breast Cancer Subtype Tested	Test Method	Sample Type	Scoring	Companion Diagnostics	Manufacturer	FDA-Approved Drugs
PD-L1	Advanced HR-negative, HER2-negative	IHC	FFPE	CPS = number of PD-L1$^+$ tumor cells plus the number of PD-L1$^+$ immune cells (lymphocytes and macrophages only), divided by the total number of tumor cells, multiplied by 100	PD-L1 IHC 22C3 Pharm Dx	Dako North America, Inc	Adjuvant pembrolizumab with chemotherapy (nab-paclitaxel, or paclitaxel, or gemcitabine plus carboplatin)
MSI/d-MMR	Any	IHC/PCR	FFPE	MSI testing evaluates for the presence of additional peaks in microsatellites of tumor in comparison to nonneoplastic tissue dMMR is determined by loss of IHC labeling for MMR proteins, MLH1, PMS2, MSH2, MSH6	Any FDA-approved antibody platform. No companion diagnostic is available at present		Pembrolizumab

(continued on next page)

Table 2
(continued)

Marker	Breast Cancer Subtype Tested	Test Method	Sample Type	Scoring	Companion Diagnostics	Manufacturer	FDA-Approved Drugs
TMB	Any	NGS	FFPE	High TMB is > 10 mutations/ megabase of genome tested	FoundationOne CDx	Foundation Medicine, Inc	Pembrolizumab

Abbreviations: CPS, combined positive score; dMMR, mismatch repair protein deficiency; FFPE, formalin-fixed paraffin-embedded; HR, hormone receptor; MSI, microsatellite instability; NGS, next-generation sequencing; PCR, polymerase chain reaction; PD-L1, programmed death-ligand 1; TMB, tumor mutation burden.

Table 3
Biomarker characteristics for single-gene alterations

Marker	Breast Cancer Subtype Tested	Test Method	Sample Type	Companion Diagnostics	Manufacturer	FDA-Approved Drugs
PIK3CA mutations	HR-positive, HER2-negative	PCR	Blood for circulating tumor DNA or FFPE	therascreen PIK3CA RGQ PCR Kit	QIAGEN GmbH	Alpelisib
		NGS	Blood for circulating tumor DNA	FoundationOne Liquid CDx	Foundation Medicine, Inc	
		NGS for somatic and germline detection	FFPE	FoundationOne CDx	Foundation Medicine, Inc	Alpelisib
BRCA1/BRCA2 germline and somatic mutations	Any	Germline testing by PCR and Sanger sequencing	Blood	BRACAnalysis CDx	Myriad Genetic Laboratories, Inc	Olaprib Talazoparib
NTRK fusions	Secretory carcinomas	NGS	FFPE	FoundationOne CDx	Foundation Medicine, Inc	Larotrectinib

Abbreviations: FFPE, formalin-fixed paraffin-embedded; HR, hormone receptor; NGS, next-generation sequencing; PCR, polymerase chain reaction.

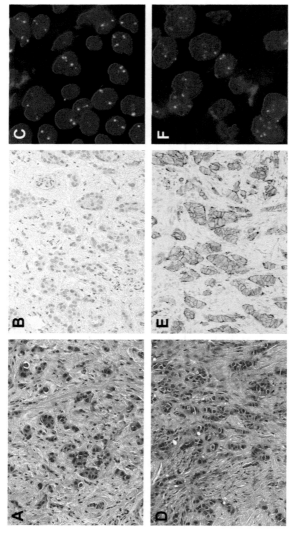

Fig. 1. Tumoral HER2 heterogeneity within a pleomorphic lobular carcinoma. Most of this primary invasive lobular carcinoma displays classic morphology with uniform cells arranged singly and in nests. (A, hematoxylin-eosin [H&E], original magnification ×200). This classic component is negative for HER2 protein overexpression by IHC (B, original magnification ×200) and is negative for HER2 amplification by FISH, with a HER2:CEP17 ratio of 1.6 and a HER2 copy number of 2.3 signals per cell (C; green = CEP17, red = HER2 locus). However, a subset of this tumor is pleomorphic, with enlarged and variably sized nuclei (D, H&E, original magnification ×200). This pleomorphic component is equivocal (IHC 2+) for HER2 overexpression by IHC (E, ×200) and is positive for HER2 amplification by FISH, with a HER2:CEP17 ratio of 4.4 and a HER2 copy number of 8.7 signals/cell (F; green = CEP17, red = HER2 locus). Tumoral HER2 heterogeneity could result in disparate biomarker profiles in different metastatic sites, or clonal expansion and predominance of biomarker profile.

Two notable independent prospective studies, the Breast Recurrence In Tissues Study (BRITS) and DESTINY studies, evaluated the changes in ER, PR, and HER2 expression in the primary tumor and any subsequent recurrences, both locoregional and distant metastases. A pooled analysis of the 2 studies' data by Amir and colleagues[8] showed that the overall discordance rates for the 3 markers were 12.6%, 31.2%, and 5.5%, respectively. Among the 3 markers, expression of PR was more often discordant than ER and HER2. The trend in the PR expression discordance was often a conversion from a positive to a negative result. This decrease or loss of PR is relevant (**Fig. 2**), because it can signal poorer response to antihormonal therapy.[9]

The discordance is explained by a wide variety of factors, including tumor biology (eg, tumor heterogeneity, clonal evolution), preanalytical variables (eg, tissue fixation, method of staining), and analytical variables (eg, subjectivity of scoring, interobserver variability). The current NCCN and American Society of Clinical Oncology (ASCO) guidelines recommend retesting all new metastatic breast cancers for ER, PR, and HER2 status. Retesting is especially important when the markers were previously unknown, initially negative, or not overexpressed. The conversion of hormone receptors and HER2 from negative to positive expression is the most clinically significant. In the analysis of Amir and colleagues,[8] 13% of hormone receptor-negative and 5% of HER2-negative primary tumors gained expression of the biomarkers in their respective metastatic tumor foci. Biomarker discordances contributed to change in therapy in approximately 14% of the patients enrolled in the 2 studies.[8] Retesting offers a subset of patients an additional treatment option with endocrine therapy, CDK 4/6 inhibitors, and/or trastuzumab.[10] Patients with discordant ER and HER2 results due to biomarker conversion tend to have worse survival than those with concordant biomarker results.[11]

Testing Techniques

ASCO and College of American Pathologists (CAP) jointly developed guidelines for the interpretation and reporting of ER, PR, and HER2 in breast cancer. As of this writing, the most recent updates to the guidelines for ER/PR and HER testing occurred in 2020 and 2018, respectively.[12,13] ER and PR testing are routinely performed by IHC. The latest guidelines recommend classifying tumors with an ER labeling of 1% to 10% as "ER low positive." These tumors more closely resemble basallike breast cancers in histology, molecular profile, and response to neoadjuvant chemotherapy than ER-positive breast cancers. The data on the benefit of endocrine therapy in this group are limited and potentially low. However, these patients are still eligible to receive endocrine therapy.[12] Cases with less than 10% ER labeling and those close to the threshold require a laboratory-specific standard operating procedure such as a second pathologist to review the score to ensure reproducibility.

HER2 assessment can be performed by IHC, FISH, CISH, or silver in situ hybridization (SISH). Although IHC is commonly used as first line for its quick turnaround time and cost-effectiveness, any approved method of testing may be used for first-line testing. An equivocal result is reflexed to a different testing method to provide a definitive result. The algorithms for the interpretation of hormone receptor and HER2 expression in metastatic tumors are the same as those for primary tumors, and guidelines are available for free online from the CAP.[14,15]

Challenges and Practical Considerations

Although specific IHC assays for ER and PR are not formally designated as FDA-approved companion diagnostic tests, in practice they function as companion diagnostics to deem patients as candidates for endocrine therapy. On the other hand, there are specific FDA companion diagnostic tests for HER2, as detailed in **Table 1**.

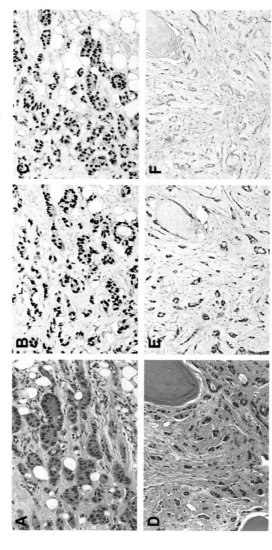

Fig. 2. PR discordance between a primary and metastatic tumor to bone in a decalcified specimen. This primary invasive ductal carcinoma (*A*, H&E, original magnification ×200) is diffusely and strongly positive for estrogen receptor (ER) (*B*, original magnification ×200) and PR (*C*, original magnification ×200). However, although biomarker testing on the patient's metastatic tumor in the iliac crest bone (*D*, H&E, original magnification ×200) shows concordant ER expression (*E*, original magnification ×200), the PR is discordant with negative (0%) labeling (*F*, original magnification ×200). Absence of biomarker labeling in a decalcified specimen could reflect true discordance, or a false-negative result due to the decalcification process.

The most common distant site of breast cancer metastasis is the bone.[16] Biomarker expression testing in this setting is particularly challenging due to the confounding effects of decalcification on antigenicity and DNA integrity in bone specimens. Rapidly acting, strong acid buffers such as hydrochloric acid lower the antigenicity of the tumor cells and frequently produce false-negative results in hormone receptor and HER2 expression results by IHC (see **Fig. 2**), as well as false-negative amplification of *HER2* by FISH.[17] Weaker acid buffers containing acetic acid and formic acid and chelating agents such as EDTA[18] are currently more widely used. Although they are slow acting, their use improves antigen preservation and stability. Bone fragments should be separated out from soft tissue in these specimens to minimize the amount of tissue subjected to decalcification. Biomarker testing can also be performed on cytology specimens, which have results comparable to core biopsies.[19]

Key points Box 1: Estrogen receptor, progesterone receptor, and human epidermal growth factor receptor-2 testing in metastatic breast cancer

1. ER, PR, and HER2 should be retested on all new metastases due to the possibility of discordance and potential management changes.

2. ER-low positive is a new category of tumors with 1% to 10% ER labeling; patients are eligible for endocrine therapy but are less likely to benefit from it.

3. Decalcification with strong acid buffers can cause false-negative results for ER, PR, and HER2 expression; this is mitigated but not eliminated with agents containing EDTA and weaker acids.

4. When sampling and grossing metastatic tumors in bone, the soft tissue fragments should be separated out to avoid decalcification of the entire tumor and to improve biomarker assessment.

PROGRAMMED DEATH-LIGAND 1 TESTING FOR IMMUNOTHERAPY
Clinical Relevance

Immunotherapy has shown a long-lasting, durable treatment response in various tumor types. Triple-negative breast carcinoma (TNBC) and HER2-positive carcinoma often display brisk tumor-infiltrating lymphocytes (TILs), reflecting a host antitumor immune response.[20] The checkpoint inhibitor pembrolizumab targeting the programmed death 1 (PD-1) receptor recently gained regular FDA approval for both high-risk early (regardless of programmed death-ligand 1 [PD-L1] status) and locally advanced unresectable or metastatic TNBC (for PD-L1+ disease); this reflects a major advance for an aggressive breast tumor subtype for which few targeted therapies are available. For advanced PD-L1+ TNBC, pembrolizumab in combination with several chemotherapeutic options (nab-paclitaxel, or paclitaxel, or gemcitabine plus carboplatin) is endorsed by the FDA.[21] Notably, the use of atezolizumab in combination with nab-paclitaxel demonstrated clinical activity in randomized phase 3 clinical trials of advanced TNBC[22]; however, the accelerated approval for its use in this setting was voluntarily withdrawn by the sponsor in 2021. Of note, the FDA also granted full approval for the addition of pembrolizumab to standard neoadjuvant chemotherapy, followed by pembrolizumab monotherapy, for high-risk early-stage TNBC regardless of PD-L1 expression.[23]

Testing Techniques

IHC for PD-L1 is used to identify patients with metastatic TNBC who are eligible for checkpoint inhibition with pembrolizumab. As of this writing, there is one FDA-approved companion diagnostic assay for the use of pembrolizumab in TNBC (see **Table 2**). To guide the use of pembrolizumab in the advanced disease setting, the PD-L1 status of a tumor is determined by the combined positive score (CPS), which is the number of PD-L1$^+$ tumor cells plus the number of PD-L1$^+$ immune cells (lymphocytes and macrophages only), divided by the total number of tumor cells, multiplied by 100. A tumor is considered PD-L1 positive, and the patient eligible for pembrolizumab, when the CPS score is 10 or more (**Fig. 3**). The only FDA-approved PD-L1 companion diagnostic that uses the CPS scoring system is the PD-L1 IHC 22C3 pharmDx assay ("22C3 assay"). For high-risk early-stage TNBC, the addition of pembrolizumab to standard neoadjuvant chemotherapy is a treatment option regardless of PD-L1 status, so PD-L1 testing to determine eligibility for neoadjuvant immunotherapy is not recommended.[23]

For the clinical trials and during the accelerated approval period for atezolizumab with nab-paclitaxel, the PD-L1 status of a breast tumor was determined by the immune cell (IC) score, which is the percentage of the tumor area occupied by PD-L1$^+$ immune cells (TILs, plasma cells, neutrophils, eosinophils, and macrophages). A tumor was considered PD-L1 positive, and the patient eligible for atezolizumab, when the IC score was 1% or greater (see **Fig. 3**). The PD-L1 companion diagnostic that used the IC scoring system was the Ventana PD-L1 (SP142) assay ("SP142 assay"). The indication for atezolizumab in advanced TNBC was voluntarily withdrawn by the sponsor in 2021.

Challenges and Practical Considerations

PD-L1 testing currently should only be performed on tumor samples from patients with locally advanced or metastatic TNBC, and only upon request from the oncologist. The PD-L1 22C3 IHC assay can be performed on both newly obtained metastatic tumor samples and archival primary tumors. Exploratory biomarker analyses from patients on clinical trials with atezolizumab showed that the likelihood of a positive PD-L1 result does vary between the primary and metastatic tumor, as well as between different metastasis niche sites. In general, metastases tend to have fewer TILs than primary tumors, decreasing the chances of having immune cells present to express PD-L1. In addition, metastases to the liver and brain tend to have fewer TILs than metastases to other sites such as the lung.[24] It is not known if this extends to PD-L1 expression as determined by the 22C3 assay. Given the totality of the data, it is preferable to avoid PD-L1 testing on liver samples if possible. Of note, the PD-L1 IHC assays are not validated for decalcified bone specimens, cytology cell blocks or smears, or circulating tumor cells.

Unlike chemotherapy, which causes well-recognized cytotoxic side effects, immunotherapy causes a spectrum of immune-related adverse events (irAEs), affecting various organ systems. Pathologists need to be aware of and recognize the histopathology of irAEs across organ types, including dermatitis, thyroiditis, hepatitis, colitis, and potentially fatal pneumonitis.[25]

Key Points Box 2: Programmed death-ligand 1 testing in metastatic breast cancer

1. PD-L1 testing is currently indicated for patients with locally advanced or metastatic TNBC

2. The 22C3 assay uses the CPS scoring system to determine patient eligibility for pembrolizumab plus chemotherapy for advanced TNBC

3. The CPS score is the total number of PD-L1$^+$ cells (tumor cells plus mononuclear immune cells), divided by the total number of tumor cells, multiplied by 100, with a positivity cutoff in breast cancer of 10 or more.

4. PD-L1 testing can be performed on either new metastatic tumor biopsies or archival primary tumor samples.

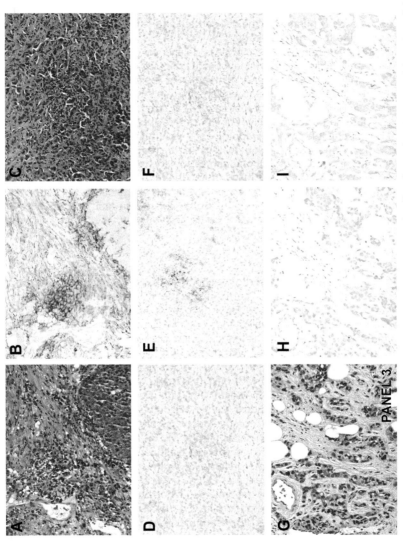

Fig. 3. PD-L1 immunohistochemistry: the PD-L1 IHC 22C3 pharmDx assay. PANEL 1: A locally advanced, primary TNBC (A, H&E, original magnification ×200) is PD-L1 positive by the 22C3 assay, with a CPS of 10 or more (B, original magnification ×200). This patient is eligible for pembrolizumab plus approved chemotherapy. PANEL 2: The archival primary tumor of a patient with metastatic TNBC (C, H&E, original magnification ×200) is PD-L1 negative by the 22C3 assay, with a CPS less than 10 (F, original magnification ×200). This patient is not eligible for pembrolizumab.

MISMATCH REPAIR PROTEIN DEFICIENCY, MICROSATELLITE INSTABILITY, AND TUMOR MUTATION BURDEN TESTING

Clinical Relevance

Some tumor types have higher tumor mutation burden (TMB) than others. Mutations accumulate in tumors by various mechanisms, including mutations (germline or somatic) in genes involved in repair of DNA base pair mismatches (mismatch protein [MMR] proteins) or double-strand DNA breaks (*BRCA1/2*). As mutations accumulate, tumor cells express new antigens on the cell surface and can become highly immunogenic and susceptible to immunotherapy.[26]

The prevalence of mismatch repair protein deficiency (dMMR) in breast cancer ($\sim$2%) is significantly lower than that in cancers of the colon ($\sim$15–20%) and endometrium ($\sim$20–30%). dMMR testing and microsatellite instability (MSI) testing have become standard of care in colon and endometrial carcinomas, whereas their use in breast cancers is limited. dMMR breast cancers are frequently high grade, associated with high TILs, and often negative for PR expression.[27] A high TMB is seen in about 5% of breast cancers, which predominantly includes TNBC and metastatic tumors. Among metastatic tumors, high TMB is more frequently seen in metastatic lobular carcinoma than metastatic ductal carcinoma. These tumors are also associated with high TILs and *BRCA1/2* germline mutations (**Fig. 4**).[28]

Single-agent pembrolizumab is now approved for any advanced solid tumor with MSI-high status, dMMR, or high TMB. Pembrolizumab is the first drug to be ever approved based on biomarkers across all tumor types (ie, a "tumor agnostic" approval).[29]

Testing Techniques

MMR testing in breast cancer is based on techniques that have been widely used in colorectal and endometrial cancers. The most commonly used testing methods are IHC or polymerase chain reaction (PCR). IHC assays for MMR proteins, namely MLH1, PMS1, MSH2, and MSH6, evaluate for loss of nuclear expression in the tumor cells. MSI is formally assessed by PCR to look for the presence of additional peaks in microsatellites in the tumor compared with normal nonneoplastic tissue. The tumors that are microsatellite unstable are further classified based on the number of unstable markers as MSI low (1 marker) and MSI high ($\geq$2 markers). In April 2021, the FDA approved the MMR IHC assay VENTANA MMR RxDx (Roche) as companion diagnostic for selecting endometrial cancers for dostarlimab-gxly immunotherapy.[30] At present, there are no MMR or MSI companion diagnostics for breast cancer. Any FDA-cleared assay may be used to determine eligibility for immunotherapy; however, this may change in the future, as new companion diagnostics are developed.[30,31]

TMB is determined either by whole-genome or whole-exome sequencing, or by sequencing targeted regions of the genome. TMB is defined as the total number of somatic mutations in a megabase of the genomic sequence analyzed. Tumors with 10 or more mutations per megabase of the genome are generally accepted as having high TMB. Unlike MSI and MMR testing, TMB testing has a companion diagnostic assay, the FoundationOneCDx assay (Foundation Medicine, Inc) (see **Table 2**), which is often required to determine patient eligibility for single-agent pembrolizumab.

Challenges and Practical Considerations

Studies on dMMR and MSI in breast cancer have shown some major drawbacks to MMR IHC in breast cancer: (1) IHC for MMR proteins shows significant heterogeneity within the tumors, which can be particularly problematic in small biopsies, and (2) loss

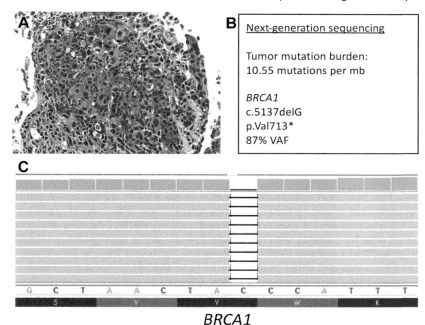

BRCA1

Fig. 4. BRCA1 mutation in a TNBC with high tumor mutation burden. This TNBC metastatic to the brain (*A*, H&E, original magnification ×200) underwent next-generation sequencing (NGS). NGS revealed a high tumor mutation burden of 10.55 mutations per megabase (Mb) (where high TMB is ≥ 10 mutations per Mb) and a pathogenic *BRCA1* mutation (*B*, *C*). The *BRCA1* mutation was previously identified as a germline change. In the tumor, this mutation has a variant allele frequency (VAF) of 87%, which is consistent with loss of heterozygosity (LOH), and biallelic inactivation of *BRCA1* in the tumor. High TMB makes the patient eligible for single-agent pembrolizumab, and the germline *BRCA1* mutation (with LOH in the tumor) makes the patient eligible for PARP inhibitors.

of MMR proteins by IHC does not correlate well with MSI testing by PCR in breast cancer. Thus, the 2 testing methods (IHC and PCR) cannot be used interchangeably in breast cancer, unlike what is done in colon or endometrial cancer. Loss of MMR proteins by IHC is more frequent than MSI.[32] At present, there are no breast cancer-specific testing guidelines for dMMR and MSI testing.

Assessment of TMB can be particularly useful in metastatic TNBC. Testing is largely driven by the oncologist in circumstances in which there are no other satisfactory treatment options available. However, because MSI and TMB are included in most next-generation sequencing assays performed for actionable mutations, this information will be available for any tumor subjected to broad sequencing.

Key Points Box 3: Mismatch repair protein deficiency, microsatellite instability, and tumor mutation burden testing in metastatic breast cancer

1. dMMR, MSI high, and TMB high are uncommon findings in breast cancers; however, TMB is seen in 5% of breast cancers and merits assessment on metastatic tumors with limited therapy options.

2. dMMR IHC testing and MSI PCR testing are not interchangeable in breast cancer.

3. Pembrolizumab is the first tumor-agnostic PD-L1 inhibitor for use in advanced tumors that are dMMR, MSI-high, or TMB-high, irrespective of tumor type.

SINGLE-GENE ALTERATION TESTING FOR TARGETED THERAPY
BRCA 1 and BRCA 2

BRCA1 and *BRCA2* are tumor suppressor genes whose protein products repair double-strand DNA breaks by homologous recombination. Approximately 10% of breast cancers have mutations in one of these genes. About two-thirds of them are germline, whereas the rest are somatic.[33,34] There are some key differences between breast cancers that arise in carriers of *BRCA1* versus *BRCA2* mutations. *BRCA1*-mutated breast cancers are often TNBC, metaplastic carcinomas, or medullary pattern and have high nuclear grade and TILs (see **Fig. 4**). *BRCA2*-mutated cancers are often of luminal immunophenotype and with variable histologic patterns and grades.[35]

Poly(adenosine diphosphate-ribose) polymerase (PARP) inhibitors (olaparib and talazoparib) and platinum-based chemotherapies are effective in patients with *BRCA1/2*-mutated breast cancers. In breast cancer, PARP inhibitors are currently approved only for patients with metastatic breast cancer and *germline* mutation in either gene.[36] In contrast, PARP inhibitors are approved for use in patients with ovarian carcinoma and either *germline or somatic BRCA1/2* mutations. Recent trials have shown that PARP inhibitors are also effective in patients with breast cancer and somatic *BRCA1/2* mutations, which, if approved, would expand the population of eligible patients.[37] *BRCA* testing not only offers a targeted therapeutic option to patients but also helps identify family members who may be at risk, and *BRCA* testing is initiated by the treating oncologist. The companion diagnostic assay is BRACAnalysisCDx (Myriad Genetic Laboratories, Inc), which uses Sanger sequencing and multiplex PCR to detect various *BRCA* mutations (see **Table 3**). This assay is currently only intended to detect germline mutations.

PIK3CA

Most (70%) breast cancers are hormone receptor positive and HER2 negative. The first line of treatment of these cancers, whether primary or metastatic, is endocrine therapy to suppress the tumor's estrogen-dependent growth. In the metastatic setting, CDK4/6 inhibitors are also considered first line in ER-positive, HER2-negative cancers (no additional testing except ER positivity required). However, about half of these patients will eventually develop resistance to endocrine therapy. One strategy to overcome the resistance is by inhibiting the PI3K/AKT/mTOR pathway components, which regulate cell functions such as growth, division, and survival. About 40% of hormone receptor-positive and HER2-negative tumors harbor activating mutations in *PIK3CA* (**Fig. 5**). At present, *PIK3CA* inhibitor alpelisib, in combination with selective estrogen receptor downregulator fulvestrant, is a second-line therapy in patients with metastatic breast cancer who have progressed on endocrine therapy with or without CDK4/6 inhibitors.[38] The treating oncologist initiates *PIK3CA* testing. There are 3 companion diagnostic assays available to detect *PIK3CA* mutations: therascreen *PIK3CA* RGQ PCR Kit (PCR test), FoundationOne Liquid CDx assay (NGS test), and FoundationOne CDx assay (NGS test) (see **Table 3**).[39] The first 2 assays can be performed on patients' blood samples using circulating tumor DNA. *PIK3CA* is the only biomarker in breast cancer that has been approved for detection in the blood through circulating tumor DNA.[40–42]

NTRK Testing

NTRK inhibitors (larotrectinib and entrectinib) are newly developed targeted therapies for solid tumors with fusions involving genes of the *NTRK* family, independent of tumor

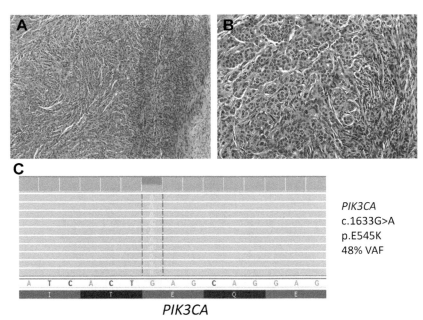

PIK3CA
c.1633G>A
p.E545K
48% VAF

PIK3CA

Fig. 5. *PIK3CA* mutation in an ER⁺ breast carcinoma. Sections of an ovarian tumor (*A*, H&E, original magnification ×100) reveal nests of uniform cells (*B*, H&E, X200) that are diffusely ER⁺ (not shown), consistent with a metastasis from the patient's known breast primary. Next-generation sequencing revealed a pathogenic *PIK3CA* mutation (*C*) with 48% variant allele frequency (VAF). The p.E545K mutation is one of the most common activating mutations in *PIK3CA* commonly detected in breast carcinoma. This *PIK3CA* mutation makes the patient eligible for *PIK3CA*-targeted therapy.

histology.[43,44] In the breast, secretory carcinomas are a rare tumor type accounting for less than 0.15% of all invasive breast cancers. These tumors are characterized by unique histology with intracellular and extracellular eosinophilic secretions, typically TNBC phenotype, and a pathognomonic *ETV6-NTRK3* gene fusion (**Fig. 6**). These tumors are identical to their counterparts in the salivary gland, thyroid, and skin.[45] Most of these tumors are indolent, whereas a small subset is aggressive with late recurrences and may benefit from *NTRK* inhibitors.

NTRK testing is unique because it is triggered by the pathologist upon histologic diagnosis of secretory carcinoma rather than by the treating clinician. Until recently, *NTRK* fusions were detected by molecular methods such as FISH and NGS. Now, a pan-*NTRK* IHC stain is available, and the *ETV6-NTRK* fusion causes a nuclear localization of the fusion protein and nuclear labeling with IHC. Diffuse and/or at least focally strong nuclear labeling with IHC has good sensitivity (83%) and specificity (100%) in detecting the *ETV6-NTRK3* fusion in secretory carcinomas of the breast.[46] IHC may be a valuable and cost-effective screening tool for secretory carcinomas, but it is not an approved companion diagnostic and molecular testing is required to confirm gene rearrangements in tumors in which *NTRK* inhibitors are being considered. The approved companion diagnostic for *NTRK* analysis is the next-generation sequencing platform FoundationOne CDx assay (see **Table 3**).[47] *NTRK* analysis is typically part of large next-generation sequencing platforms and will be assessed in all breast cancer subtypes submitted for sequencing. However, the

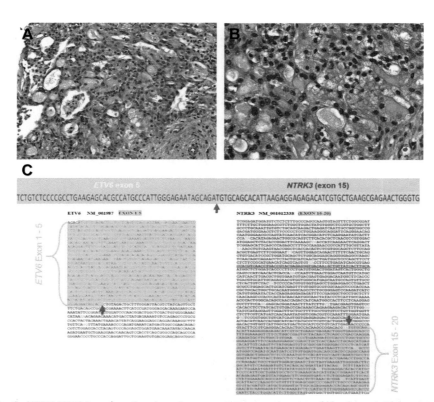

Fig. 6. NTRK-ETV6 translocation in primary secretory carcinoma of the breast. This primary breast carcinoma displays cribriform architecture (*A*, H&E, original magnification ×200), uniform nuclei, and eosinophilic luminal secretions (*B*, H&E, original magnification ×400), suggesting secretory carcinoma. Targeted gene sequencing confirms the presence of a translocation between *ETV6* exons 1 to 5 and *NTRK* exons 15 to 20 (*C*), confirming the diagnosis of secretory carcinoma. If the patient were to develop metastatic disease, the presence of the *NTRK-ETV6* translocation would make the patient eligible for *NTRK*-targeted therapy.

vast majority of breast cancers known to have *NTRK* alterations are secretory carcinomas.[48]

Key Points Box 4: Single mutation testing in metastatic breast cancer

1. Patients with germline *BRCA1/2* mutations and metastatic breast cancer are eligible for therapy with PARP inhibitors

2. Patients with somatic *PIK3CA* mutations in ER-positive, HER2-negative metastatic breast cancer are eligible for targeted therapy with alpelisib

3. Patients with *NTRK* rearrangement metastatic breast secretory carcinomas are eligible for targeted therapy with larotrectinib and entrectinib

4. Although *NTRK* assessment can be performed on any breast cancer subtype, there is no utility in testing nonsecretory carcinomas.

5. IHC to detect NTRK protein is an effective screening and diagnostic tool in secretory carcinomas, but molecular confirmation is required for treatment with NTRK inhibitors.

FUTURE DIRECTIONS
Novel Assays

Liquid biopsies of blood for circulating tumor DNA (ctDNA) is a time- and cost-effective, noninvasive method for obtaining tumor material for testing. Liquid biopsies have a unique advantage of capturing tumor heterogeneity within a single tumor site and across multiple metastases. ctDNA testing can be used to detect new actionable genetic alterations in tumors that progress, to measure tumor burden, and to monitor tumor relapse or metastasis.[49] Two of the most common single-gene alterations detected by testing ctDNA are *PIK3CA* and *ESR1,* both relevant therapeutically.[50] At present, the only FDA-approved companion diagnostic assay that uses ctDNA in breast cancer is for detecting *PIK3CA* for treatment with alpelisib. All other uses of ctDNA in breast cancer remain experimental at present.

Emerging Biomarkers

The presence of TILs is both a prognostic and predictive biomarker in breast cancer.[51,52] Society-level guidelines for scoring and reporting TILs and clinical guidelines for meaningful use of this information will be required before TILs can be incorporated into clinical practice.

Another big challenge in the interpretation of biomarkers is interobserver and intraobserver variability. Image digitization and image analysis technologies may provide reproducible, objective, and accurate assessment of biomarkers, as platforms are validated and approved for clinical use.[53] Finally, novel anti-HER2 therapeutic agents such as antibody drug conjugates have shown beneficial responses even in HER2 nonamplified breast cancers in clinical trials, leading to a proposed new category of breast tumors, "HER2-low."[54] Future testing algorithms may see inclusion of this category to identify tumors that respond well to emerging anti-HER2 agents.

SUMMARY

Metastatic breast cancers remain a challenge to treat. However, the landscape of testing and therapeutics in these cancers is evolving rapidly. As new targeted therapeutics are developed, corresponding companion diagnostic assays are also being developed to determine which patients will benefit from these therapies Sequencing platforms are a cost-effective tool to comprehensively gather genomic information on multiple biomarkers simultaneously to guide therapy. It is important for the practicing pathologist to be aware of biomarker recommendations and testing platforms to effectively participate in and guide the multidisciplinary care of patients with metastatic breast cancer.

DISCLOSURE

G. Jagannathan: None; M.J. White: None; R.R. Xian: None; L.A. Emens: honoraria from AbbVie, Amgen, Celgene, Chugai, GCPR, Gilead, Gritstone, MedImmune, Peregrine, Shionogi, and Syndax; honoraria and travel support from AstraZeneca, Bayer, MacroGenics, Replimune, and Vaccinex; travel support from Bristol Myers Squibb, Genentech/Roche, and Novartis; potential future stock from Molecuvax; institutional support from AbbVie, Aduro Biotech, AstraZeneca, the Breast Cancer Research Foundation, Bristol Myers Squibb, Bolt Therapeutics, Compugen, Corvus, CyTomX, the US Department of Defense, EMD Serono, Genentech, Maxcyte, Merck, the National Cancer Institute, the NSABP Foundation, SU2C, Silverback, Roche, the Translational Breast Cancer Research Consortium, Takeda, Tempest, and HeritX; royalties from

Aduro Biotech; A. Cimino-Mathews: Research grants to institution from Bristol-Myers Squibb; consultancy/honoraria to self from Bristol-Myers Squibb and Roche.

REFERENCES

1. Female breast cancer — cancer stat facts. Available at: https://seer.cancer.gov/statfacts/html/breast.html. Accessed January 2, 2021.
2. NCCN Clinical Practice Guidelines in Oncology (NCCN Guidelines): Breast Cancer. NCCN.org. 2021. Available at: https://www.nccn.org/guidelines/category_1. Accessed April 26, 2021.
3. Jørgensen JT, Hersom M. Companion diagnostics-a tool to improve pharmacotherapy. Ann Transl Med 2016;4(24). https://doi.org/10.21037/atm.2016.12.26.
4. U.S. FDA. Developing and labeling in vitro companion diagnostic devices for a specific group of oncology therapeutic products guidance for industry. FDA guidance documents. 2020. Available at: https://www.fda.gov/vaccines-blood-biologics/guidance-compliance-regulatory-information-biologics/biologics-guidances. Accessed April 25, 2021.
5. U.S. FDA. List of Cleared or Approved Companion Diagnostic Devices (In Vitro and Imaging Tools). 2021. Available at: https://www.fda.gov/medical-devices/in-vitro-diagnostics/list-cleared-or-approved-companion-diagnostic-devices-in-vitro-and-imaging-tools. Accessed April 28, 2021.
6. Allott EH, Geradts J, Sun X, et al. Intratumoral heterogeneity as a source of discordance in breast cancer biomarker classification. Breast Cancer Res 2016;18(1):1–11.
7. Jabbour MN, Massad CY, Boulos FI. Variability in hormone and growth factor receptor expression in primary versus recurrent, metastatic, and post-neoadjuvant breast carcinoma. Breast Cancer Res Treat 2012;135(1):29–37.
8. Amir E, Clemons M, Purdie CA, et al. Tissue confirmation of disease recurrence in breast cancer patients: pooled analysis of multi-centre, multi-disciplinary prospective studies. Cancer Treat Rev 2012;38(6):708–14.
9. Bardou VJ, Arpino G, Elledge RM, et al. Progesterone receptor status significantly improves outcome prediction over estrogen receptor status alone for adjuvant endocrine therapy in two large breast cancer databases. J Clin Oncol 2003;21(10):1973–9.
10. Van Poznak C, Somerfield MR, Bast RC, et al. Use of biomarkers to guide decisions on systemic therapy for women with metastatic breast cancer: American Society of Clinical Oncology clinical practice guideline. J Clin Oncol 2015;33(24):2695–704.
11. Hoefnagel LDC, Moelans CB, Meijer SL, et al. Prognostic value of estrogen receptor α and progesterone receptor conversion in distant breast cancer metastases. Cancer 2012;118(20):4929–35.
12. Allison KH, Hammond MEH, Dowsett M, et al. Estrogen and progesterone receptor testing in breast cancer: ASCO/CAP guideline update. J Clin Oncol 2020;38(12):1346–66.
13. Wolff AC, Elizabeth Hale Hammond M, Allison KH, et al. Human epidermal growth factor receptor 2 testing in breast cancer: American society of clinical oncology/college of American pathologists clinical practice guideline focused update. J Clin Oncol 2018;36(20):2105–22.
14. Estrogen and progesterone receptor testing in breast cancer guideline update. American Society of Clinical Oncology/College of American Pathologists; 2020. Available at: https://www.cap.org/protocols-and-guidelines/cap-guidelines/

current-cap-guidelines/guideline-recommendations-for-immunohistochemical-testing-of-estrogen-and-progesterone-receptors-in-breast-cancer. Accessed April 19, 2021.

15. HER2 testing in breast cancer. American Society of Clinical Oncology/College of American Pathologists; 2018. Available at: https://www.cap.org/protocols-and-guidelines/cap-guidelines/current-cap-guidelines/recommendations-for-human-epidermal-growth-factor-2-testing-in-breast-cancer. Accessed April 26, 2021.

16. Chen MT, Sun HF, Zhao Y, et al. Comparison of patterns and prognosis among distant metastatic breast cancer patients by age groups: a SEER population-based analysis. Sci Rep 2017;7(1):1–8.

17. Clark BZ, Yoest JM, Onisko A, et al. Effects of hydrochloric acid and formic acid decalcification on breast tumor biomarkers and HER2 fluorescence in situ hybridization. Appl Immunohistochem Mol Morphol 2019;27(3):223–30.

18. van Es SC, van der Vegt B, Bensch F, et al. Decalcification of breast cancer bone metastases With EDTA does not affect ER, PR, and HER2 results. Am J Surg Pathol 2019;43(10):1355–60.

19. Pareja F, Murray MP, Jean RD, et al. Cytologic assessment of estrogen receptor, progesterone receptor, and HER2 status in metastatic breast carcinoma. J Am Soc Cytopathol 2017;6(1):33–40.

20. Cimino-Mathews A. Tumor-in filtrating lymphocytes and PD-L1 in breast cancer (and, what happened to medullary carcinoma?). Diagn Histopathol 2021;1–7.

21. Cortes J, Cescon DW, Rugo HS, et al. Pembrolizumab plus chemotherapy versus placebo plus chemotherapy for previously untreated locally recurrent inoperable or metastatic triple-negative breast cancer (KEYNOTE-355): a randomised, placebo-controlled, double-blind, phase 3 clinical trial. Lancet 2020; 396(10265):1817–28.

22. Schmid P, Adams S, Rugo HS, et al. Atezolizumab and Nab-paclitaxel in advanced triple-negative breast cancer. N Engl J Med 2018;379(22):2108–21.

23. Schmid P, Cortes J, Pusztai L, et al. Pembrolizumab for early triple-negative breast cancer. N Engl J Med 2020;382(9):810–21.

24. Cimino-Mathews A, Ye X, Meeker A, et al. Metastatic triple-negative breast cancers at first relapse have fewer tumor-infiltrating lymphocytes than their matched primary breast tumors: a pilot study. Hum Pathol 2013;44(10):2055–63.

25. Michot JM, Bigenwald C, Champiat S, et al. Immune-related adverse events with immune checkpoint blockade: a comprehensive review. Eur J Cancer 2016;54: 139–48.

26. Fusco MJ, West HJ, Walko CM. Tumor mutation burden and cancer treatment. JAMA Oncol 2021;7(2):316.

27. Cheng AS, Leung SCY, Gao D, et al. Mismatch repair protein loss in breast cancer: clinicopathological associations in a large British Columbia cohort. Breast Cancer Res Treat 2020;179(1):3–10.

28. Barroso-Sousa R, Jain E, Cohen O, et al. Prevalence and mutational determinants of high tumor mutation burden in breast cancer. Ann Oncol 2020;31(3):387–94.

29. Marabelle A, Fakih M, Lopez J, et al. Association of tumour mutational burden with outcomes in patients with advanced solid tumours treated with pembrolizumab: prospective biomarker analysis of the multicohort, open-label, phase 2 KEYNOTE-158 study. Lancet Oncol 2020;21(10):1353–65.

30. U.S. FDA. FDA grants accelerated approval to dostarlimab-gxly for dMMR endometrial cancer. Drug approvals and databases. Available at: https://www.fda.gov/drugs/drug-approvals-and-databases/fda-grants-accelerated-approval-dostarlimab-gxly-dmmr-endometrial-cancer. Accessed April 26, 2021.

31. Venetis K, Sajjadi E, Haricharan S, et al. Mismatch repair testing in breast cancer: The path to tumor-specific immuno-oncology biomarkers. Transl Cancer Res 2020;9(7):4060–4.

32. Fusco N, Lopez G, Corti C, et al. Mismatch repair protein loss as a prognostic and predictive biomarker in breast cancers regardless of microsatellite instability. JNCI Cancer Spectr 2018;2(4). https://doi.org/10.1093/jncics/pky056.

33. Winter C, Nilsson MP, Olsson E, et al. Targeted sequencing of BRCA1 and BRCA2 across a large unselected breast cancer cohort suggests that one-third of mutations are somatic. Ann Oncol 2016;27(8):1532–8.

34. Nik-Zainal S, Davies H, Staaf J, et al. Landscape of somatic mutations in 560 breast cancer whole-genome sequences. Nature 2016;534(7605):47–54.

35. Sønderstrup IMH, Jensen MBR, Ejlertsen B, et al. Subtypes in BRCA-mutated breast cancer. Hum Pathol 2019;84:192–201.

36. Robson M, Im S-A, Senkus E, et al. Olaparib for metastatic breast cancer in patients with a Germline BRCA mutation. N Engl J Med 2017;377(6):523–33.

37. Tung NM, Robson ME, Ventz S, et al. TBCRC 048: phase II study of olaparib for metastatic breast cancer and mutations in homologous recombination-related genes. J Clin Oncol 2020;38(36):4274–82.

38. André F, Ciruelos E, Rubovszky G, et al. Alpelisib for PIK3CA-mutated, hormone receptor–positive advanced breast cancer. N Engl J Med 2019;380(20):1929–40.

39. Martínez-Saéz O, Chic N, Pascual T, et al. Frequency and spectrum of PIK3CA somatic mutations in breast cancer. Breast Cancer Res 2020;22(1):1–9.

40. U.S. FDA. FDA approves first PI3K inhibitor for breast cancer. Available at: https://www.fda.gov/news-events/press-announcements/fda-approves-first-pi3k-inhibitor-breast-cancer. Accessed April 26, 2021.

41. U.S. FDA. FDA approves liquid biopsy NGS companion diagnostic test for multiple cancers and biomarkers. Available at: https://www.fda.gov/drugs/fda-approves-liquid-biopsy-ngs-companion-diagnostic-test-multiple-cancers-and-biomarkers. Accessed April 26, 2021.

42. U.S. FDA. FDA approves alpelisib for metastatic breast cancer. Available at: https://www.fda.gov/drugs/resources-information-approved-drugs/fda-approves-alpelisib-metastatic-breast-cancer. Accessed April 26, 2021.

43. Scott LJ. Larotrectinib: first global approval. Drugs 2019;79(2):201–6.

44. Al-Salama ZT, Keam SJ. Entrectinib: first global approval. Drugs 2019;79(13):1477–83.

45. Diallo R, Schaefer KL, Bankfalvi A, et al. Secretory carcinoma of the breast: a distinct variant of invasive ductal carcinoma assessed by comparative genomic hybridization and immunohistochemistry. Hum Pathol 2003;34(12):1299–305.

46. Harrison BT, Fowler E, Krings G, et al. Pan-TRK immunohistochemistry. Am J Surg Pathol 2019;43(12):1693–700.

47. U.S. FDA. FDA approves companion diagnostic to identify NTRK fusions in solid tumors for Vitrakvi. Available at: https://www.fda.gov/drugs/fda-approves-companion-diagnostic-identify-ntrk-fusions-solid-tumors-vitrakvi. Accessed April 25, 2021.

48. Remoué A, Conan-Charlet V, Bourhis A, et al. Non-secretory breast carcinomas lack NTRK rearrangements and TRK protein expression. Pathol Int 2019;69(2):94–6.

49. Canzoniero JVL, Park BH. Use of cell free DNA in breast oncology. Biochim Biophys Acta 2016;1865(2):266–74.

50. Buono G, Gerratana L, Bulfoni M, et al. Circulating tumor DNA analysis in breast cancer: Is it ready for prime-time? Cancer Treat Rev 2019;73:73–83.

51. Tan PH, Ellis I, Allison K, et al. The 2019 World Health Organization classification of tumours of the breast. Histopathology 2020;77(2):181–5.
52.. Tan PH, Ellis I, Allison K, et al. World Health Organization Classification of Tumours: breast tumors. 5th editionVol 2. Lyon, France: IARC Press; 2019.
53. Dermawan JK, Mukhopadhyay S, Shah AA. Frequency and extent of cytokeratin expression in paraganglioma: an immunohistochemical study of 60 cases from 5 anatomic sites and review of the literature. Hum Pathol 2019;93:16–22.
54. Tarantino P, Hamilton E, Tolaney SM, et al. HER2-low breast cancer: pathological and clinical landscape. J Clin Oncol 2020;38(17):1951–62.

Moving?

Make sure your subscription moves with you!

To notify us of your new address, find your **Clinics Account Number** (located on your mailing label above your name), and contact customer service at:

Email: journalscustomerservice-usa@elsevier.com

800-654-2452 (subscribers in the U.S. & Canada)
314-447-8871 (subscribers outside of the U.S. & Canada)

Fax number: 314-447-8029

Elsevier Health Sciences Division
Subscription Customer Service
3251 Riverport Lane
Maryland Heights, MO 63043

*To ensure uninterrupted delivery of your subscription, please notify us at least 4 weeks in advance of move.

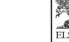

9780443182945